LONGING HEART
Empty Arms

ISBN: 978-1-60920-057-2
Printed in the United States of America
©2013 by Sally M. Jones

Library of Congress Cataloging-in-Publication Data

All scripture references used are from the
New American Standard Bible. Anaheim: Foundation, 1997.

Ajoyin Publishing, Inc.
PO Box 342
Three Rivers, MI 49093
www.ajoyin.com

Please direct your inquiries to admin@ajoyin.com

LONGING HEART
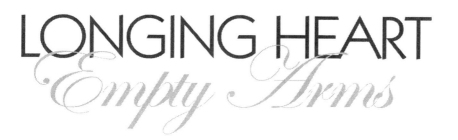

♥ ♥ ♥

Sally M. Jones

Ajoyin Publishing, Inc.
www.ajoyin.com
1.888.273.4569

Introduction and Acknowledgments

I have always enjoyed writing and sometimes in the back of my mind would contemplate writing a book, but I always just pushed the thought away and figured I would "get to it" sometime during my adult life. Sometime during 2008 is when I really began feeling a strong tug to write. A particular story came to me and I had a sudden and nearly overwhelming urge to write it. I did begin working on it some that year, but put it off after awhile. This urge and tug I was feeling grew and grew until I thought about writing every day. It turned into a dream of mine to write and publish Christian fiction novels. More and more stories kept coming to me. So in late 2008 I began to write down all of my ideas. That first novel that had come to me kind of got pushed into the background and my passion turned towards one of the stories that had come to me: the journey two women go through together through infertility. I was experiencing infertility personally and felt God had brought that to the forefront because He wanted me to write it while it was fresh in my mind. So I started the book in January of 2009 and worked on it only a few times within a month or two. Then I didn't make time for writing as I should and at times procrastinated, and got busy with life and eventually received my miracle . . . my positive pregnancy test. Then I was busy being a stay at home mommy to my sweet girl after she was born in April of 2010. But my husband and I began talking about my dream to write again and my husband helped me come up with a plan to give me the house to myself to have time to write. I decided to buckle down and get serious this time. I had written scenes so many times in my head to other books or this one, come up with more story ideas, etc. and I was ready to finish this book. So in April of 2011 I got serious and wrote once or twice a week (other than a couple breaks from various things) until I finished in June of 2012. My son was born July 31st and after I had some time to adjust to our family of four, I completed the editing process and then began the publishing process in early October. So it's been a long work in progress and a long time coming!

There are so many people I would like to thank for a number of reasons!

Thank you and I love you to all of my family and my friends (both on the Internet and in "real life").

Thank you, mom and dad for raising me to be the woman I am today and for bringing me up in the Lord to the best of your ability. I love you both!

Thank you to my dear friends Bethany Jacobs and Lisa Sparks Carpenter who have been my friends for years. I appreciate you encouraging me and praying for me about my writing dream before many people even knew about it.

I also would like to give a big thank you to my dear "Internet friend" Ashley Yancey. You have really been there for me the past several years and especially through this journey through infertility and I appreciate it more than I could ever express. She also gave me the idea for what I wanted to be the title of this book. We were talking one day and she said something like "Even if God never gives me biological children, it's like He's shown me that He will give me heart children." And some of my other internet friends had told me that you could have a mother's heart even if you are not yet a mother. So I came up with "The Heart of a Mother." I was not able to use that as my title, but it resounded so much with me that I chose to use it to wrap up the book. I consider you one of my closest friends, Ash, and you are part of the reason I knew my main characters could have such a bond. I still can't believe we have gotten to be pregnant together not once, but twice! God is so good!

A big thank you to all my "internet friends"; a group of

women whom I have become very close to over the years. I have poured my heart and soul out to you girls and you couldn't have been more sweet or wonderful. I appreciate you always listening, your friendship, prayers, love for me, and helping more than you could ever possibly know! Thank you to all of you who helped me through infertility (you know who you are!). A special thanks to those who I continue to be in close contact with and who continue to be amazing friends to me through the mundane and big things in life: Amber H., Ashley C., Ashley Y., Brieanne R., Danielle K., Jenny S., Katie H., Katie T., Kellie S., Leanne G., Melissa ("Mel") C., Melissa O., and Melissa R. You girls have known more details than any one as I wrote this book and prayed me through and I appreciate that so much! I love you all!

Thank you to all the great girls from my online TTC group for your advice, listening ears, seemingly unending knowledge, and amazing support! It was so awesome to have people I could always turn to with questions, to give an update to, or to vent who completely understood me.

A special thanks also to my dear friend Bethany Jacobs and my sister-in-law Abby Jones for being my pillars of support while we went through infertility. Beth you knew from day one and I appreciated having someone to open up to that whole time! It was nearly a year in I believe when you found out "on accident" Ab, but your help was invaluable! Thanks to you both for just listening to me and letting me get things off my chest, crying with me, and always being there when I needed to vent. I appreciate your words of comfort, your prayers, your support, and for always being there for me and loving me through. I can't imagine how difficult it must be to try to support someone when you want so badly to help but know you can't and when you don't always know what to say. But you helped more than you'll ever know and I love you both dearly.

Thank you to all of you who knew about this at some point throughout the journey before we shared it with everyone and encouraged and prayed for us. You know who you are and I thank you from the bottom of my heart.

I also want to say thank you to my parents for watching Jenna for me most of the nights I worked on writing. Also thank you to my mother and father-in-law for keeping Justin and Jenna company a few times while I worked. You all helped me immensely by allowing me to have the house to myself so I could have the quiet to concentrate and write.

Thank you mom for helping me edit by looking for inconsistencies in my time line, spelling errors, or letting me know if something didn't flow right. I know you have great attention for details and you helped me catch and fix things I wouldn't have otherwise noticed. Thanks so much for all your hard work!

Thank you also to my Aunt Pam and Sherry Gilmore for all your help in the publishing process.

To my husband and I's families: Thank you all for loving us and supporting us. We are glad we get to go through life with you all and enjoy spending time with all of you. You are all near and dear to our hearts! We love you Tom and Cathy Jones; Jason and Abby Jones and our sweet nieces Nevaeh and Livia; Dan and Jen Affriseo and our sweet niece and nephew Sophia and Daniel; Bill and Jenny Curtis; and Luke Curtis.

Thank you, Lord, for giving me the blessing of all my family, friends, and loved ones and all the other numerous blessings in my life. I know my desire to write is from You and I pray that I bring You honor and glory from it.

I also want to specifically mention two of my greatest blessings from my heavenly Father. First, my pot of gold at the end of the rainbow, my sweet daughter Jenna Mae. Daddy and I say all the time how worth the wait you were and how perfect you are to make up for our time of waiting. We love you more than words could ever express! I feel like the Grinch; my heart is always expanding to fit all the love I have for you in it. Secondly, to my sweet little son Jayden. We had chosen your name years earlier, even before our journey through infertility. Fittingly, your name means "God has heard." You arrived shortly after I finished writing

4

this book. Once again, my heart seemed to expand to fit all my love for you in it. Daddy and I feel immensely blessed to have you in our lives, little man. Thank you, God, for my amazing little miracles.

And last, but certainly not least, I want to say a huge thank you to my dear husband, Justin. Thank you for loving me unconditionally with all of your heart and being my biggest supporter in everything I do, including my writing. Thank you for believing in me and encouraging me to keep going. You are my perfect match, my soul mate, and I'm so glad I had you by my side while we struggled through infertility. I know it only made us stronger and I thank God for you every day. I'm so glad I have you by my side through all the ups and downs of life. I love you with all my heart, sweety!

Dedicated to all who have gone or are going through infertility.
You are close to my heart and in my thoughts and prayers.

"He makes the barren woman abide in the house
As a joyful mother of children.
Praise the LORD!"
Psalm 113:9

Prologue

November 2004

Jadie and Chase Taylor both sat cross-legged on their bed with a Bible spread open between them. This was the day they had been waiting for! They had been married for almost exactly two and a half years. Their desire for children had grown seemingly from the moment they said, "I do." But they wanted to have some time just for the two of them, since they were young, before they began trying to start a family. They also had wanted to get a home of their own instead of renting before taking the plunge into parenthood. They had purchased their first home about six months ago. It was somewhat small, one story, but cozy; and nestled just off a country road with a small yard and trees surrounding the area. It had three bedrooms, one and a half bathrooms, a decent sized kitchen and dining area, and a homey living room with a small fireplace.

They had been planning this specific day for nearly six months. They had thought, talked, and prayed about it ever since they purchased their home. And this is the date they had decided on. November 17th, 2004. Jadie was nearly giddy with excitement and Chase's eyes practically danced. They both smiled hugely at each other. The fact that they were getting ready to start trying to make a baby together made them both so happy. This day was probably only second to their wedding day. Jadie, unaware that Chase was doing the same thing, allowed her mind to wander back to that beautiful day. It was May 4th, 2002 and the weather couldn't have been better. They were married outside at a relative's home surrounded by flowers, beautiful decorations, and loved ones. It was a somewhat simple, but elegant and beautiful ceremony. It couldn't have been more perfect. Jadie saw flashes of them all done up for the day with the rays of the sun splashing down on them and almost dancing as if they were as happy as the bride and groom. She could see herself and Chase experiencing the ceremony and sharing their vows, holding hands and walking and laughing together, greeting guests, enjoying their outdoor reception at sunset, and a hundred other quick memories of the day. Jadie blinked and allowed herself to come back to the present. Chase was looking right at her and they both laughed at how they had allowed their minds to wander. Chase picked up the Bible again and asked if they could read a few more passages about parenting. Jadie nodded fervently and waited as he turned the pages in the Bible she had owned since High School. The pages were somewhat yellowed and there were passages that were underlined, circled, and highlighted, and notes at the bottoms of some of the pages. But she loved the familiarity of that Bible and sighed contentedly as she put her hands behind her to support herself and leaned back, waiting for Chase to begin reading again.

After he had read a few more passages, they scooted closer together, held hands, and talked about their dreams for their children. What they would look like, what their personalities would be like, what their names would be, and on and on. After only a moment of silence Jadie sat up a little straighter and said to Chase, "You know, I think it's the most amazing thing how God created everything to work. How we make babies by making love, what more beautiful way could there be? And then, that baby that we make together is the perfect picture of marriage and the oneness we share. It is both of us combined into one little person. I just think that's a miracle." Chase smiled. He loved when Jadie was that sincere and shared her heart with him like that. He agreed it was a beautiful thing indeed. He leaned forward and gently kissed her nose before suggesting that they pray together. They did just that. Asking that God would bless them and that they would be pregnant soon if that was His will, that the pregnancy would go well and they would have a healthy baby, and that He would lead and direct them and help them to be the parents and spiritual leaders they needed to be. Chase said "Amen" and Jadie chorused it. Then he rose and shut the curtain on the still light sky and the snow floating steadily down outside. He carefully set the Bible on the nightstand, laid on the bed, and scooted closer to Jadie. She smiled and lay down next to him. They just held each other and shared more of their hearts with one another. After saying "I love you" to each other, Chase looked into Jadie's face and got that mischievous grin that Jadie loved. He tried to sound serious as he said, "Now. Let's get to that beautiful part we were talking about earlier." Jadie giggled before the sound of her voice was muffled with his kisses.

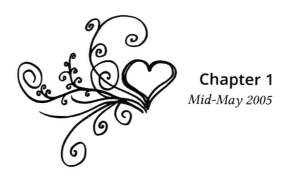

Chapter 1
Mid-May 2005

J adie Taylor paced back and forth in her bathroom. How long could three minutes last? It felt like she'd already been doing this for an hour. She grabbed the pink box off of the counter and stared at it again. She sighed and threw it back down and resumed her pacing. Chase would be home from work in two hours. Wouldn't it be wonderful to be able to give him the news he so desperately wanted to hear? And that she so desperately wanted to be true? The familiar creak of the boards beneath her feet when she stepped in certain spots strangely comforted her, even if only slightly. She stared at the clock for the tenth time in the past few minutes. She suddenly remembered being a little girl walking down a hospital hallway with her father. She hadn't eaten enough that day and hospitals had a strange effect on her. She had felt as though she would pass out. Her legs had felt like they weighed one thousand pounds apiece and it took all she had to drag them to keep up with her. That's what the second hand on the clock seemed to be doing now. It would seem to hold still, drag, then finally tick over to the next second. She wiped her sweaty hands up and down on her jeans and then tucked the stray hairs that weren't long enough to fit in her ponytail behind her ears. She wanted this so badly she could taste it. The closer it came to finally being able to look at the little white stick sitting on the sink's counter top that she was so desperately trying to avoid peeking at, the more nervous and excited she got at the same time. Her hands trembled slightly and her pulse seemed to continue to increase by the second. She could feel her heartbeat pulsating through different parts in her body and also hear the strange sound that slightly vibrated in her ears. *Please God, let it be positive.* She glanced at the clock again. *It's almost time*, she thought. She allowed her mind to wander, if only to keep her sanity for the last remaining moments she had to wait.

Six months. It had been six long months since she and Chase had begun trying to conceive their first baby. The first few months it was somewhat easier to shrug it off. "This is normal," they must have told each other one hundred times. But this month she had felt herself becoming worried. When would it happen? Why was it taking so long? Was something wrong with her? With Chase? With both of them? She tried to not let the thoughts consume her, but it was difficult. Both sets of their parents had no trouble getting pregnant at all. In fact, she used to chuckle when Chase's mother would tell her, "Your father-in-law and I could hang our underwear on the line near each other and get pregnant." Her parents had conceived herself and her younger brother within the first cycle or two of trying. So why was this becoming so difficult for her and Chase? Could something really be wrong? She had tried to make the negative thoughts, feelings, and worries go away, but she couldn't seem to overcome them. And now this month she had hope. Her breasts had been tender for a few days and she was so sleepy all day she could hardly stand it. She was making more trips to the restroom with each passing day and even had nausea, especially in the mornings. So this had to be it! Didn't it?

Jadie took a deep breath and made herself stand a little straighter. *Don't let yourself over think this Jadie*, she thought. *You are going to work yourself into a frenzy. Nothing is wrong with either of you! Everything is perfectly fine. In fact, you'll probably see two pink lines at any moment now.* She felt her heart slow down just a bit and relaxed some. She blew out her breath and literally sagged with relief. Then the next thought caused her pulse to pick up again, *No, no! You cannot get your hopes up that much either! Just calm down! What will be, will be. God is in control.* She walked to the toilet and sank down onto the closed lid and placed a hand on each side of her head, cradling it. She put her elbows on her knees and bent over slightly. Why did she have to put so much pressure on herself? It would be okay, even if she wasn't pregnant. She swallowed and realized that wasn't completely true. This whole process was beginning to get to her. *Dear Lord, please help me! I hardly know what to say right now.* She stole a peak at the clock and her heart thundered into an irregular rhythm. It was time. *Please be with me as I look at these results. Help me not to be too disappointed if it is negative. Help me to see that You know everything and this will happen for us in your timing.* She took a deep breath again. *Give me strength Lord. Amen.* She stood up and straightened herself to full height. She still didn't look right away. She just needed a moment to gather herself. She kept taking deep breaths. In and out, nice and slow. Yes, that was helping. She glanced at the clock again just to be sure she had waited sufficient time. She walked the few small steps over to the sink and faced it. She looked at herself in the mirror. How haggard she looked! She could almost see the worry etched on her face. Why was this so hard? *You can do this. Just look down, Jadie. Remember, God is in control. Everything will be fine.* She forced herself to smile slightly into the mirror. She felt a burst of strength and bravery in herself and forced her eyes down to the counter top where the test lay. So much was resting on such a little item. Her eyes reached the pregnancy test and her heart nearly stopped in her chest. She stood frozen, unable to move for a moment. And then she leaned closer to make sure she had interpreted it right. *How can this be? That's impossible!* She grabbed the box she had tossed down earlier and ripped it open and drug the directions back out. She hastily scrambled over to the light switch and turned it on. The sky had been growing darker and she hadn't even noticed. Her hands trembled violently as she tried to find the right page. She forced her eyes to read the words and then looked at the diagram, then back at the test, and back at the diagram. It was as she thought. She sighed deeply and just continued to stare at the test. Maybe if she stared harder . . . no. The reality of the situation hit her like a ton of bricks. She placed her hands on the counter top to stable herself. She felt the tears well up in her eyes. So much had been resting on that test! She had prayed that she would accept the results no matter what they were. But she was failing miserably. She felt as though her heart plummeted to her stomach and the tears began to slide down her cheeks. She looked at the test again, her vision so blurry she could barely see it. There it was: screaming at her. How would she tell Chase? How could she tell him that she'd given in and taken the pregnancy test and that there was only one pink line? Negative. Never had that one word seemed more final and terrible than today.

She tried not to allow it, but the tears came faster. She couldn't lie to herself. She wanted to be a mommy more than anything in this world. And even though it had only been six months, that test had crushed her dreams. Her heart felt broken. And right at that moment, she knew nothing would comfort her. The world around her grew darker as the snow began to fall quickly outside. She had to get out of this bathroom. Suddenly, it felt as though hours had passed and she felt very drained. She angrily threw the test into the wastebasket and walked out and into their kitchen and dining area. She pulled a chair out and sank into it. She dropped her face into her hands and allowed the tears to come more freely now. She looked up again for a moment and out the window. It was practically a blizzard out there. And it seemed it was nearly dusk for how much the sky had grown dark. None of this improved her mood. Cold and dark indeed. Just like her heart.

♥ ♥ ♥

Chase was more than relieved when he pulled into the driveway after work. It had gotten dark much earlier than normal today and the snow was coming down very fast. *How odd to be having such a storm in May*, he thought. This was the first time that had happened here in Wisconsin in possibly decades. He got out of the car and immediately began to be covered in the snow. He saw the kitchen light was on. Such a warm sight to come home to. It made him feel better before he even walked into the door. Jadie had the day off today, so he hoped she had started dinner. He reached the door, which had a slight overhang, and brushed the snow off of his sleeves and stomped his work boots on the cement step to free them from the clinging snow. He stepped inside and immediately rubbed his gloved hands together. He still couldn't believe they had their own home. He loved the feeling of owning something and having something he could call his own. He and Jadie were very happy here and the fact that they would soon have a baby living in this house made him even more excited. He glanced around their home from where he stood. There was a small area of linoleum beneath his feet with a rug on it. Ahead of him and slightly to the left was where the hallway began that led to two of the bedrooms and a full bathroom. He was standing in an open area and the kitchen was directly to his right. It had an "L" shape of counter tops with cupboards above them and a large gap in between. On the other side of that was their small dining area where they had a table and chairs. From that position, you could look out of their glass sliding door. The view was a small area of yard, then the trees that lay between the home and the road. In front of him and slightly off to the right was the living room that was spacious and cozy. Off to the right, in the center of the open area that contained the living room, kitchen, and dining area, was the hallway that led to their bedroom that contained a half bathroom as well. Their bedroom sported one very large window that looked out into their back yard. He sighed with contentment and smiled. Even though it had been a year, he still was so proud of their home.

He came out of his musings and wondered where that sweet little wife of his was. Many days, especially if she hadn't worked that day, Jadie would meet him at the door. He took his jacket off and hung it on the coat rack to his left and placed his gloves inside the pocket. He walked around the kitchen area to where their dining area was. Jadie was sitting at the table. She didn't seem to notice him at first, but finally turned around to face him and looked up at him. She seemed sad and distracted. This was very unlike his wife who was usually a very happy person. Chase walked over to her and kneeled on the floor in front of her. He searched her eyes hoping they would give him some indication of what was going on with her. He placed his hands on her thighs and said in a concerned and soft voice, "What's wrong, sweetheart?" Her beautiful green eyes welled up with tears and she pressed her lips together. A sure sign that she was very upset, but trying not to give into all the tears that she really wanted to. She shook her head back and forth just slightly. He sat up a little more and took her into his arms. He hated it when she cried. She was so precious to him and it hurt his heart to see those tears streaming down her face. He felt her body jerk slightly now and then and she attempted to stifle her sobs. "Aww, honey. What is it? Please tell me." He held her a little tighter and rubbed her back while he waited for her to regain control. Finally she backed away from him, her face wet with tears, and slightly scrunched up as she still struggled to not cry. "Well . . . you know how I was having all of those symptoms?" His mind raced. Yes, she had been having a lot of pregnancy symptoms. What on earth could this be about? He nodded and rubbed his hands up and down her arms. "Yes, baby, I remember." She wiped some of the tears from her face and hesitated. "Gosh, this is so hard!" she choked out before placing her forearm over both of her eyes. She sniffed and took some shaky breaths. "Well, I know I said I wasn't going to test at least until my period was a week late, but I had so many symptoms that I couldn't wait any longer." He tucked some stray hair behind her ear, caressed the side of

her face, and tried to calm his heart that was now racing. "Okay
... go on." Her shoulders literally sagged. "It was negative, Chase.
Negative. How can that be?" And her tears began again. "Oh
baby, I'm so sorry" he said as he pulled her into his arms once
again. He was trying to be brave for her, but inside, his heart had
plummeted and he felt so sad and disappointed. He wanted to be
a daddy so badly. And he knew how badly Jadie wanted a baby.
She would be an amazing mother; he had absolutely no doubt
about that. He sighed. Was it normal for it to take this long? What
if something was wrong with him and he couldn't give Jadie her
children? He stiffened at the thought. *You cannot think like that.
Everything will be fine. Sure, she had some symptoms this month,
but it wasn't meant to be. It will happen soon. We just have to be
patient.* He felt his resolve strengthen slightly. But his poor wife.
She was so loving, tenderhearted, and sweet. He knew this must
be crushing her. *Lord, please help this not to be so hard on her. Give
her Your comfort, Your strength.* He took Jadie's arms and gently
pushed her away from him a bit. Her tears had slowed, as if
she was relieved to just finally have said the words to him. He
looked her in the eye and said, "Sweety, it will be okay. I know
it's hard! I know we both want a baby more than anything in
this world. But God is with us. And it will happen soon, I just
know it will. We just have to try to be patient. I know you're
hurting and that's very understandable; I am too! But we just
need to keep trying and it'll happen, you'll see." Her eyes had
gotten intent on him while he was speaking. He hoped he had
said the right thing. She finally spoke with resignation in her
voice, "I know, honey. It's just so disappointing. I really thought
I was this time, ya know?"

"I do, baby, I do. But it's alright. It'll happen, you'll see." She
hugged him again briefly and then got up and walked around
and into the kitchen. He followed her and for the next half
hour, they prepared dinner together and talked more about the
situation. His heart hurt for his wife and for himself, really. He
understood her desire for a child. By the time dinner was well

under way, he was happy to see that Jadie's tears had subsided and that while still a bit down, she was doing much better. He smiled at her as they continued to talk, but he thought *I hope this doesn't take much longer.*

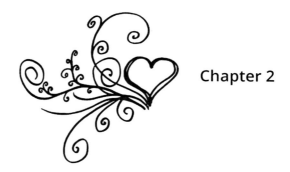

Amy Whitley sighed loudly as she scrubbed the dishes extra hard. She and her husband Jake were fighting . . . again. As she stewed and willed herself to remain angry, she noticed Jake had quietly left the room and went into their bedroom. She suddenly stopped washing the dishes and stared out the window of their modest home in Wyoming. She felt the anger begin to dissipate in her chest and she blew out a long breath, causing a wisp of hair to blow straight in the air and then fall against her cheek. Why did it seem like lately that every week or two they had to have a fight? They both were stressed and on edge and seemed to take it out on each other. She also knew another reason. The thing that seemed to loom over them every day even though they tried to pretend it wasn't there. The fact that they had been trying for just over two years to have a baby, but it wasn't working. They had starting seeing a fertility specialist three months ago, but so far, they couldn't find what was wrong. She knew that the worry, stress, expense, and everything else tied up in that entire situation was getting to them. They had left it in God's hands, but why was it still so difficult? She resumed doing the dishes again, but the fight in her had left her. She now felt badly for fighting with Jake. She knew all of the stress, wondering, and waiting was beginning to affect their marriage. Even though having a baby meant the world to them, she had the sudden realization that they could not let it ruin their relationship with each other. Because if damage had been done, it wouldn't magically go away simply because they got pregnant. And then what kind of parents would they be to their children if they were fighting all the time and no longer had a good relationship?

She had made up her mind and turned the water back on. She would finish the dishes and then speak with Jake immediately.

♥ ♥ ♥

Jake sat on the edge of the bed in he and Amy's bedroom with no light on. His forearms rested on his thighs and his hands were clasped together, his right foot gently bouncing up and down. His eyes were fixed on a spot on the wall and he stared unblinking as he was deep in thought. Why did he and Amy let things escalate like that? He knew they were both stressed, but he adored Amy more than anything in the world and absolutely hated when they were at odds with one another. Since they were no closer to finding an answer in the baby department, it could be months or years until they had a child. They couldn't allow things to continue this way or they would only get worse.

He hated the pressure he felt right now. He was working on getting his license to be an electrician so that he could make a better life for him and Amy, and God willing, their future children. It was more difficult than he'd imagined and working at least forty-five hours a week on top of his studying and training didn't help matters.

Added to that were the feelings of inadequacy for not being able to give his wife a child. It made him feel like less of a man. Of course, the doctor had been focusing on Amy right now, but next week he had to give a sperm sample so they could see if he was a factor in things as well. He realized that Amy's cycles were not always regular and that it could be her, but for some reason, he still felt responsible. In a way, he wanted it to be him as well because he loved Amy too much to wish the feelings of not being whole on her. He took a deep breath and blew it out slowly for a long time. God would get them through and He had a plan in all of this. He knew it and believed it with his entire being. But knowing that didn't take away all the feelings that came along with something like this.

But he could not let things affect Amy and him like this. After all, they were working together through life, and in trying to make a child together. And they were taking everything out on each other. The irony of that thought had not hit him before that moment. They were supposed to be working through these things together, as God intended, but instead they were battling against each other every time things got hard.

He knew Amy was upset with him, but he also knew they would talk things out before they went to bed. They always did.

Jake was still deep in thought when he heard Amy enter the room behind him. He had left the light in the bedroom off, but the light in the hallway was on and cast a bit of light on the wall in front of him. He didn't turn to glance at her. Not because he was still angry or didn't want to see her, but he just felt resigned and very tired. At that moment he felt as though the weight of the world was on his shoulders and on top of it all, he and Amy were fighting which always made him feel incomplete and not right.

She slowly crossed the distance between them and sat next to him on the bed. He knew by the sigh that escaped her that she was feeling much the same way as he was. He turned his head towards her just slightly so he could see her out of the corner of his eye and then turned his head back. That quick glance told him that she was no longer angry either.

He felt slightly better from the moment he heard her slightly deep voice come out in a very gentle, almost quiet tone. "I'm sorry, Jake." She reached over and placed her hand on top of his.

Jake blew out his breath. "So am I, Amy. So am I."

They sat for another moment in silence before Amy continued gently, "You know what I realized out there?"

Jake looked up at her and she realized that was encouragement to continue.

"If we fight and hurt our marriage now because we want a baby, what will happen when the baby comes? We'll finally have what we wanted so desperately, but in the process of getting there we will have destroyed us. Doesn't that kind of defeat the whole purpose? Kind of ironic, isn't it?" She made a small huffing sound and folded her hands in her lap and looked back to the wall in front of them.

Jake nodded silently before replying in a soft and gentle tone of his own, "I was thinking the same thing. I realize we're stressed Amy. I know this isn't how we imagined things would go. We got excited, we made plans, and we began the wonderful process of starting our family . . . of making a baby. But months turned into more months, which turned into years." Jake watched in surprise as Amy's body went rigid and tears welled up quickly in her eyes and spilled down her cheeks. His wife was a very strong woman and was not prone to crying very often. He softened his voice even more and took her hand again, "I know you're hurting." Even though Amy knew that with Jake she could never hold her tears, especially when he used that soft, sweet voice that he was now and on top of that the feel of his hand in hers; she looked at him anyways. What she saw there caused her tears to fall faster. His face was pinched with agony and his eyes were filled with pain and desperation. His voice reflected that desperation as he continued, his voice almost strained and sounded somewhat like a hoarse whisper, "And it's killing me. Killing me, Amy. I love you and I can't . . . " he paused for a minute and Amy nearly gasped as she watched his eyes mist with tears. Something she'd only see happen a handful of times in the entire time she'd known him which was most of their lives. His voice grew even more strained and he gritted his teeth, forcing the words out, "I can't stand this. I want to give you what you want . . . what we both want. And I can't. I feel as though I'm failing you. I can't stand the pain this is causing us. We can't do this to ourselves any longer."

Tears continued to coarse down Amy's cheeks and she clung desperately to his hand, waiting for him to continue. "We know God has a plan for us and we need to trust Him no matter how much longer this takes."

How much longer this takes. Amy's eyes slid shut for a moment with the thought she always tried to avoid. That this could be a long road to answers. To a baby. Or, worst of all, that this may never happen for them. She willed herself to focus on Jake.

"I know we have been trusting Him, but we're not leaning on Him or praying about this the way we should. We need to surrender this to Him. And that's not going to make it any less painful or hard, but it may give us some peace while we wait."

Amy nodded her agreement. Tears gathered and threatened to spill over his lower lid. "I cannot and will not lose what we have together in this process. We will do this together and we will be stronger on the other side. This should be bringing us together, not trying to tear us apart. And I don't know what's going to happen or how long this will take, but we will make it. And we will love each other even more than we do right now."

Amy choked on a sob as she watched two, then three tears slide down her husband's handsome face. Jake swallowed and the desperation left his voice and his teeth became unclenched. He cleared his throat and continued in a soft tone that was still barely above a whisper, "I do not believe God would give us the desire for children and not have it fulfilled. We will be parents one day, Amy. I believe that and I want you to too. We will have our family one day. Believe that with me? Please, Amy?" His eyebrows had raised and his voice pleaded as he asked the question. He almost seemed like a little boy and her heart clenched. She could barely hold herself from sobbing aloud, but she nodded her head before reaching her arms out for him to hold her. He did so and held her tightly. She felt a few of his tears land on her shoulder, but she was practically soaking his shirt with her own. She loved this man more than life itself. He was so strong and brave. And the fact that he loved her and wanted this baby as much as she did was made abundantly clear tonight. They had always talked through their feelings about this, but they had always tried to tread lightly on the subject and even avoided it at times or tried to make light of it. But she knew they were both beyond pretending everything was going to be okay. They were realizing it might not be and they couldn't just brush it off any longer. This was serious and was affecting their lives, their hearts, their stress levels, and their marriage. It was time to surrender it all to God as Jake had said, start facing reality and continue to seriously pursue answers at the fertility specialist. It wasn't that they had avoided the topic altogether or just assumed it would all be okay, but they were going to start looking at things more realistically and dealing with things head on instead of trying to pretend it wasn't as bad as it was.

Once she felt composed enough, she shared these thoughts with Jake, still snug up against him. He agreed completely and they decided to start being more open about it and talking about it whenever either of them needed to.

"And like I said before," Jake added, his arms still wrapped tightly around Amy, "most importantly we need to start praying every day about this. We have prayed, but not like we should be. We need God's help to get through this."

Amy nodded and turned her head and snuggled against Jake's chest and nuzzled her face into his neck. He kissed the top of her head. *What a day*, Amy thought. All the stress had gotten to them and finally culminated into a fight. But she was extremely grateful for the conversation that followed. She felt much better about the future and although things may even get worse before they got better, God was with them. And she and Jake would go through it together. She felt extremely safe, loved, cherished, and comforted in her husband's strong arms. She felt very grateful for their marriage and the love they shared. And after sharing their hearts so freely with each other, there was no other place she'd rather be than right here. In Jake's arms with both of their shirtsleeves still damp from tears.

Chapter 3

J adie sat down at her computer desk in her bedroom and hit the power button on the tower. While she waited for the computer to turn on, she prayed that God would continue to heal her heart. The pain was much less than it had been on Tuesday, but she was still concerned. Trying to make a baby was becoming more difficult than she'd ever imagined it to be.

She had worked yesterday at the flower shop that was less than a ten-minute drive from their home. She worked there part time along with two women from her church and a few other women from their town. Her scheduled days varied, but she always worked three and a half days a week and every once in awhile, would cover a shift for someone on Saturday. She enjoyed working there and the eight dollars an hour she made there helped a little bit with the expenses at home. Once her taxes were taken out and she purchased gas for the following week and paid for the insurance on her car, it wasn't much, but every little bit helped.

This particular Thursday she had only worked until noon and now she wanted to see if she could find some sort of group on the Internet where other women were trying to conceive who she could talk to. She shifted slightly on the folding chair in front of the computer desk and connected to the Internet. She googled what she was looking for and browsed through some of the results. She preferred the set up of online groups to message boards, so she began going to sites that had groups and searching through their topics. She found a few groups, but many did not have very many members and not very much activity. After an hour or so of searching she stumbled across a group that seemed to have quite a few members and a lot of activity. She smiled to herself and excitedly sent the request to join.

She knew it may take awhile to be accepted by the group's moderator, so she forced herself to disconnect from the Internet and find something else to do. She remembered that she had some laundry going in the garage that was probably done by now. She switched over the loads, started a new one, and put the dried load into a basket and carried it to their bedroom. While she folded the clothes, she wondered how Chase was doing at work today. She was so proud of how hard he worked for them. He worked for a local contractor doing all types of odd jobs. He had always enjoyed being outdoors and working with his hands, so he loved his work. Still, Jadie knew the hours could be long and the labor demanding, not to mention the unpleasant weather he sometimes had to deal with. But today was a very pleasant day, the snow from two days ago melted and nearly forgotten.

The sunshine and warmth also seemed to have melted some of her pain and deep disappointment from the other day. She still felt full of questions and she was sad it hadn't happened for them yet, but some of the pain had abated. Joining this group made her happy, excited even. She was hoping she could get some tips and maybe talk to other women who had been trying for awhile. Lest she be tempted to go check the computer already, she tried to think on what else she had wanted to accomplish today. She glanced at the clock and realized it was a bit earlier than she thought. She knew she had some meat in the freezer and decided to start preparing a scrumptious crock pot meal for dinner that evening. She smiled as she headed out to the kitchen. Yes, she was feeling much more optimistic. This was a good day and she wanted to feel happy and carefree. Suddenly a verse popped into her head. It was Psalm 118:24. "This is the day which the LORD has made; Let us rejoice and be glad in it." That of course made her think of the song that she had grown up singing in church with that verse for the lyrics. She decided to go put one of her favorite "Third Day" CD's in the stereo in the living room before beginning her work on dinner. She was going to see how quickly she could finish her tasks and then maybe she'd allow herself to get online quick and see if her membership was accepted before Chase got home from work. As the music gently floated into the kitchen and to her ears and the aroma of the food already tantalized her senses, she smiled broadly. A good day, indeed.

♥ ♥ ♥

Amy decided to take a break from cleaning and her other chores and check her e-mail. She had one day off a week from her job at the library (usually Friday, like it was today) in town and she always made the most of it. But on the days she had off she also liked to take quick breaks and catch up on her e-mail from her trying to conceive group. She was able to check it in the evenings sometimes, but she usually was spending her time with Jake. So her days off were good days to catch up on the week's e-mails. She clicked on them one by one and responded to some of them where she felt she could lend encouragement or experience and offered silent prayers for some of the ladies who were really struggling. Her eyes landed on an e-mail saying they had gotten a new member. *Jadie . . . that's an interesting name; very pretty.* She read through her introduction and responded and welcomed her warmly. Then she noticed she had written another e-mail to the group. She read it and felt her heart clench. The poor thing had really started struggling with her emotions. Amy could totally relate. She also noticed how open, honest, and eager she seemed. She also couldn't help but notice she had asked for prayer. For some reason, this girl just really pulled her heartstrings and she instantly felt a connection to her. She decided to e-mail her off-list to see if there was anything she could do for her and to let her know she would keep her in her prayers.

Amy knew that she was the motherly type. She always had been. She had two younger sisters and as some had teased her in school, had always been "old for her age." She could tell Jadie was a strong woman in some ways from how she had written the lengthy e-mail. But at the same time, she seemed very tenderhearted and almost vulnerable and it instantly made the mother hen in Amy want to protect her with her wings. She said a special prayer for Jadie and then disconnected from the Internet. She still had many things on her list to accomplish today so that she could freely enjoy her weekend with Jake.

As she continued to work around the house, many of the women who were on the group frequently came to mind. Some women only posted now and then while others were on every day and tried to respond to most of the posts by the other women. Amy had once joined a message board but ended up leaving because she found there to be too much information on some other topics that interested her and it led to her spending more time on the internet than she liked. She'd never heard of groups before, but ended up hearing one of the other girls from her first message board mentioning one once. She had decided to look them up and found that instead of having many different pages and discussions, that groups tended to be focused on one thing. Their home page was set up completely different and while you could read the posts online, she selected the e-mail option. So every time someone posted on the group, it came to her e-mail. So she could easily read the posts in the order they were written and the subject line always referenced which conversation this post pertained to. Plus, people always left the text from the previous post underneath their own writing, so it made it easy to follow the conversations. She had grown to love not only the set up of the group, but had felt such a pull on her heart for the women of the group. Some of them also were Christians like her while some were not. Some women were young, some older. Some had pursued treatments while some just wanted to try natural methods and everything in between. Some women were so sweet and others were a bit rough around the edges. But they all had something in common and they all, on some level, understood each other. She made sure to pray for them all each day and for specifics on her day off when she took the most time to read through the e-mails. She tried to sometimes send a Scripture verse to some of the posters' personal e-mail off the group, to encourage some of her sisters-in-Christ. For those who didn't know the Lord, she prayed extra fervently for them, that they would come to know Him as their personal Savior.

As she opened her small closet that stored her broom, mops, cleaning supplies, and other various items in her kitchen and pulled out the broom and dust pan, she thought again of the new girl who had joined. She was fairly certain she'd never heard the name "Jadie" before. She wouldn't have been entirely sure of how to pronounce it, but Jadie had written in parenthesis next to her name: "pronounced 'Jay-dee'. Like 'Sadie' but with a 'J' instead. Just so you all know since EVERY ONE asks" followed by a smiley face. But there was just so much about her that intrigued Amy for some reason. She couldn't put her finger on it. She couldn't shake the feeling that she felt so drawn to her. She decided to pray for her again as she swept her kitchen and small entry area to the side of it. Secretly she hoped Jadie responded to her e-mail soon. She really hoped maybe they could get to know each other better off the group.

J adie was so happy she had this Friday off from work. She had been working on writing out some bills and balancing her check book. Now that she had some laundry going, she anxiously waited for her computer to boot up. She had been a part of the Trying To Conceive (abbreviated TTC) Group for a little over a week now and couldn't wait to get online and check her e-mail. Almost right away she'd received a couple of e-mails about etiquette, a few rules, and an e-mail full of TTC abbreviations and lingo. At first it was so overwhelming! She couldn't believe how many different terms and words there were for everything. Just from looking for a group to join she had figured out that "TTC" stood for "trying to conceive." At first she just skimmed the list and decided not to worry about it at the time. But as she had excitedly read her first few e-mails, she realized humorously that she was going to have to study that list as if there were an exam she was going to have to take if she was ever going to understand what was being said. She also had already timidly asked a few questions as she had never heard of some of the things these women were referencing. She had received so many responses to her introduction and she felt so welcomed right away. Her more lengthy post had also gotten so many responses from other women who said that they completely understood her and some of them had some suggestions for her. It felt so good to know she was not alone in her thoughts, feelings, and frustrations. Some women shared they'd been trying for years and others for just a couple of months and claimed they were already in worse shape than her. However, some of the suggestions overwhelmed her because there just seemed to be so many options of things to try. For now she wanted to just keep learning about some of these options and just continue the basics of trying without using any of these other helps.

While she had always understood the basics of the female body as far as reproduction, she'd already learned some interesting things about ovulation and her cycle and how all of that worked. She also saw that many of the women on the group were "veterans" at TTC and talked about infertility. She shuddered even now thinking about it. Infertility was just something she never gave much thought. She had only known one or two couples who had ever been through that and she'd never talked to them much about it. She'd heard of other people going through it as well, but she didn't know them personally. She recalled hearing people saying that so-and-so already had a couple of kids and shouldn't be using meds to get pregnant. That if God wanted them to have children, He would have made that happen. At the time she had heard those things she hadn't given it much thought. But now, hearing these women's stories and even thinking more about the couples she had known, she wondered what she would do in their shoes. It pained her to even have to think about the possibility of not being able to conceive on her own. She mentally shook her head to try to free herself from the negative thoughts. That wasn't something she even wanted to consider. Everything was fine . . . these things could take time. Several of the women on the group had already assured her that it was completely normal for a young, healthy couple to take up to a year to conceive. She felt certain after hearing that that nothing was wrong with her and Chase. *It's normal*, she thought again. She was sure it would happen any time now.

She also had been so touched to receive a very sweet e-mail from a woman named Amy. Amy had complimented her on her name, introduced herself in a bit more depth, and even shared a couple of encouraging Scriptures at the bottom. Jadie was very touched by the strength and maturity she sensed from Amy, but also her honesty in stating that she had felt drawn to her. She also was surprised by her openness. She had already seen in Amy's e-mails to others on the group that she seemed just slightly guarded. Jadie didn't blame her one bit. This all seemed very personal to be discussing with people and on the internet, no less! It was comforting to Jadie though that only people who were approved to the group could see any of the messages or other parts of the group. In some ways, it also seemed easier to talk to strangers about it. But Amy had shared some of her own struggles over the past two years. Jadie couldn't imagine trying for that long and still not even know what was going on. She felt the questions and doubts had been suffocating a couple of times and she couldn't imagine how much that must be multiplied once you were two years in. Still, Amy seemed somewhat optimistic now that they were seeing a "fertility specialist." Jadie felt nervous for Amy that they hadn't figured anything out yet. *Is it complicated to figure out what's wrong when something is?* she wondered.

She and Amy had since written back and forth a couple of times now and Jadie was struck, as Amy had admitted to being, by how strong a connection she felt to Amy. But she supposed it wasn't all that odd. She pondered on how often when she met someone in person how it seemed that they had just clicked. Chase was one of those people. She had just instantly felt comfortable with him and like she had known him for many years in a way. She smiled at the memory of the first few times she had spent time with him. She was reading her e-mails now and saw that she had another response from Amy. After reading it, she prayed for Amy and her husband, Jake; that God would bless them with a baby soon.

That reply sent, she read some more e-mails from the group.

She had to admit to herself that she had blushed on more than one occasion from some of the things she read at times. But she supposed trying to make a baby did involve some pretty personal details. One abbreviation she did not recognize and had to ask about was "CM." She must have blushed clear through to the roots of her hair when one woman responded that it stood for "cervical mucus or your discharge." One that made her smile and laugh outright, but again, also blush; was "BD" which she learned stood for "baby dance." She also had learned that "O" stood for "ovulate," "CD" stood for "cycle day," and that "BFN" stood for "big fat negative" and "BFP" stood for "big fat positive" when they took pregnancy tests. She had already been familiar with some internet lingo such as "LOL" for "laugh out loud," "DH" for "dear husband," "ttyl" for "talk to you later," and so on. But it was all this TTC lingo that she was still trying to learn. While she was thinking of it, she decided to read over the list again that had been sent to her. She didn't have the best memory and she hoped that continuing to see the terms written out in context and also going over the list occasionally would help imbed what they meant into her head. Right now most of it still felt like a foreign language and like she may never pick all of it up. But she was determined to try.

She kept her list open in another tab and continued to read through some of the other e-mails. There seemed to be a new person or two joining every few days. Some of them never posted again and Jadie wondered at times if they were just observers or just never checked back to read posts. She was already beginning to recognize some of the women's names who were on there quite often and responded to many of the posts. Amy was one of the more frequent posters and Jadie always enjoyed reading her responses. She seemed so grounded, mature, and had a wisdom about her. Jadie hoped to keep their off-list e-mails going so she could continue to get to know this fascinating woman better.

Oh, how interesting! Jadie thought as she read a post from someone mentioning that they'd put a picture of themselves on the group under "Photos." She hadn't looked at the Group's home page much and hadn't even noticed that there was a page for photos. She opened another tab and typed in the Group's address and then signed in. She saw the "Photos" link right away and clicked on it. She was surprised that there were probably twenty members who had posted pictures of themselves and pictures with their families on there. She clicked on each person's folder and it had their name and e-mail address listed. It was neat to put some faces with the names of the people she had been reading posts from. She smiled at some of those who had a child or two and their sweet family photos or those who had pets or had posted a picture of themselves making a silly face. They were in alphabetical order and she was surprised as the scrolled down to see Amy's e-mail address, which started with her last name, near the bottom. She excitedly clicked on the folder and was excited to see a wedding photo and an everyday picture taken of Amy and Jake. She clicked on each photo individually to make them larger. They were both such good photos. Jadie studied them both intently. Amy's face and frame seemed to fit what Jadie knew of her personality so well. She looked to be about medium height and was about medium build, but thin. She had short hair that just barely touched her shoulders that was dark blonde. Her eyes looked like a medium brown, but they were quite pretty. She was pretty fair skinned and her jaw was almost a bit square, but she had delicate facial features. Jadie found her to be lovely. She seemed somewhat serious, yet friendly. Jake was quite tall and broad and had black hair and very dark eyes. His face looked . . . she could think of no other words than "manly" and "strong." Yet there was a gentleness and kindness in his eyes. But it seemed clear to Jadie by their body language that both were slightly solemn, very strong people–especially Jake, but they were both also very kind. Jadie smiled and felt quite happy to have been able to get this peek into their lives and whether they were aware or not, their personalities. She would ask Chase what he thought about her posting a couple of photos and maybe she would do that soon as well.

   She glanced at the photos one more time before closing the tab. She heard the faint buzz of the dryer echo through the garage. *Perfect timing*, she thought. *Time to get back to work!*

Chapter 5

J ake sat on the slightly cold examination table at the doctor's office waiting for the doctor to come in to speak to him. He gripped the table on each side of his thighs and stared at the wall. Was he really here? Had he really just done this? It felt surreal in a way. He felt frustrated that it had come to this. Why couldn't he and Amy just make a baby the same way every other couple seemed to? Quickly and almost effortlessly.

He felt nervous too. There was nothing about a doctor's office he enjoyed. He was a private man and thinking about what he had just done and still having to have the uncomfortable conversation with the doctor soon was about enough to do him in. But here he was all the same.

Poor Amy had endured a few uncomfortable procedures by this point. And they had talked and agreed that it was time to figure out what was going on. So he was doing his part. He just hoped they got some answers soon and could move forward with the next step. What that was he didn't know yet.

Dr. Moyer, their fertility specialist, had talked to them about some of the things that could be wrong and if so how they could proceed, but he and Amy had not decided yet what they would do if any of those things turned out to be the case for them. They were still both mulling it over, praying, and really thinking about what they wanted and how far they were willing to go with all of this.

There was a time that Jake, had he been asked, would have said there was no way on earth he would ever go through anything "unnatural" to conceive a child and that included even going to the doctor for it. But that was before . . . well, before all they'd been through. He could almost picture what it would be like to have his small son that looked like him mostly but softened by some of Amy's beauty and sweetness riding around on his shoulders laughing. Or what a little girl would look like as she sleepily walked up to him and stretched out her arms and said, "Daddy" and wanted to be held. The thought was so touching to him and the desire resonated so soundly in his soul that he realized he had gotten tears in his eyes. He sat up a little straighter and forced himself to stop staring at the wall. He pinched his nose with his fingers and closed his eyes for a moment to regain control.

He wanted children so badly that he could almost taste it and yet it seemed so far out of his grasp. He scoffed inwardly at how before he would have so quickly dismissed the idea of going to the doctor for something like this. But now he wondered why he'd been so close minded and what was so wrong with wanting to know what was going on with their bodies? When something else didn't work correctly on someone's body or it didn't do something it was supposed to do no one questioned it or thought it strange if they went to the doctor to find out what was going on; so why was this any different? He knew instantly that it wasn't. Besides, sometimes he worried about Amy. She said she had known other women who had irregular cycles, but sometimes he wondered what caused it and if it could be serious to other aspects of her health. Especially since they'd been seeing Dr. Moyer and he'd heard about some of the health issues that could cause something like that.

He sighed. Yes, they were doing the right thing for them by doing this. Amy had known a couple of people on her group that were only interested in natural methods of trying to have a baby and didn't want to go to the doctor and there were some who were not willing to go to the doctor at all. She had explained some of their reasoning behind it and he completely understood. But he and Amy had talked about this. They'd waited nearly two years before doing anything and the stress was too much. They weren't willing to give up hope on having biological children, so this was the next step for them, they'd decided after pondering things in their hearts and praying both separately and together.

Jake heard the sound of a woman's voice as she laughed in the hallway. He could hear another woman as well. Obviously the two co-workers found something amusing. A shiver ran down his spine and he felt nauseated for a split moment. He couldn't help but wonder if they were talking about a patient out there . . . making fun of them. And if he was being honest, he wasn't wondering about just any patient, but he thought maybe they were talking about him. He realized he was being paranoid and ridiculous, but he couldn't help it. The thought remained. He shifted slightly on the table and the strange crackling noise of the paper beneath him seemed exceptionally loud.

When he'd called to make the appointment to have his sperm tested, he'd made it very clear on the phone to the nurse that there were to be no dirty magazines in his room. The woman seemed surprised at first, but was quick to assure him that they would make sure that nothing like that was present in his room. Amy had warned him about it from reading the e-mails on her group. Some of the other women of faith had said their husbands had walked in the room only to see pornography magazines on the table. As if it wasn't awkward enough for them, they had to personally place the magazines out of sight or request for someone to remove them. Jake knew that when the time came it would be awkward enough without having to worry about something like that. He was glad Amy had told him and he thought he had handled it. But when he arrived earlier today he felt he should make sure. So when the nurse called his name and took him to a small room, before she even could place her hand on the door knob he said he had made a request when he'd called to make his appointment and wanted to make sure it'd been followed. She'd dropped her hand that was in mid-air reaching for the door knob and then raised it to hold onto the clipboard she was holding against her chest with her other hand. "What request was that, sir?" She seemed polite, kind, and professional and although this was extremely awkward, Jake kept the walls up in his eyes and the confidence in his voice like he was good at doing and forced himself to respond, "That there would be no magazines or pictures in my room." He could tell it took the nurse a moment for this information to register and when it did, to his surprise, her eyes lit up and she smiled and fought to squelch a laugh. "Are you serious?" she said a little too loudly and then seemed to realize what she'd just said. She cleared her throat and looked down for a moment and then looked at him again and attempted to say in a more professional tone, "Are you referring to the pornography magazines, sir?"

Jake was not amused and kept his voice sure, calm, and even but stern when he replied, "Yes. I don't want anything like that at all in that room."

She blinked at him a few times and stood there as if she wasn't sure how to respond next. Jake tried to remain patient, but he felt like his frustration and fear were culminating to the point where she must be able to see his pulse beating through his skin on his neck. After what seemed like forever she placed her hand on the door knob and seemed a bit more serious and kind again and said, "Would you like me to check the room for you before you go in? I hadn't heard of the request you'd made so I can't be sure if your room is . . . was prepared the way you'd like."

He appreciated her now returned professionalism and said, "Yes, please, if you would."

He waited as she entered the small room and shut the door behind her. She was gone less than a minute and then the door re-opened and she came out and left the door ajar for him. She still had the clipboard up against her chest, but he could see the top half inch or so of two magazines sticking up above the top of the clipboard.

"There you go sir. When you are finished, place the specimen in that small door there," she turned and gestured into the room and pointed in the direction of the cubby in the wall, "and then go back up to the front desk and she'll take you to an examination room." She smiled politely and he tried to keep his voice steady as he answered "Thank you" and then quickly stepped into the room and shut the door. He still had his hand resting on it and he set his forehead there and rested it for a moment with his eyes closed.

This was just horrible and he absolutely hated it. No doubt the people in the waiting room heard that conversation since the hallway that led to a few small rooms was only a few yards away from where they sat and his was the closest room to them. He felt like a big baby for making such a big deal about what he had to do for this test. He was a grown man after all and he felt his thoughts of wanting nothing more than to flee this office and never return quite childish.

He sighed. He knew all men had to feel uncomfortable about something like this, but he felt he was taking it too far. He stood up and surveyed the small room for a moment and saw the cup sitting on the edge of the small sink for him with a label on it that had his name, birth date, and some other information. The nurse had verified his information earlier and must have placed the cup in the room while he was in the waiting area. He tried to take a few deep breaths to calm himself, but he felt his pulse racing. He was convinced he had never felt more uncomfortable in his entire life.

He took one more deep breath to steady himself and closed his eyes to pray. *Lord, please help me right now. Help this to lead to answers for Amy and I. Just please ... be with me I pray.* He didn't know what else to say. He knew Amy was at home praying too. It had seemed to give him a small boost of courage.

Now he not so patiently waited for the doctor to arrive. He wasn't sure why he even needed to see the doctor, but he was about to find out. Not thirty seconds later there was a couple light knocks on the door and a male doctor entered the room. He was a tall and lean fellow, handsome and dark haired, and his smile seemed to light up his entire face.

He reached out and shook Jake's hand heartily. "So did you survive, big guy?"

Jake liked his easy manner and didn't mind his making light of the situation. He laughed slightly and shook his head a couple of times. "I guess I did."

The doctor laughed too. After introducing themselves, the doctor let him know that he was just going to do a brief and basic physical. *Ahhh. That's why I'm wearing this ridiculous hospital gown.* He told himself.

"I see you were referred here by Dr. Moyer. She's a great Doctor. You're in good hands." He placed the cold stethoscope against Jake's chest.

"Yes, she is. Thank you." While he still wasn't thrilled to be here, he was so glad the worst part was over. And the doctor's easy manner and kindness continued to put him more and more at ease. In a few minutes he could get into his normal clothing and go home to Amy. He could hardly wait.

♥ ♥ ♥

Amy tried not to pace back and forth in the kitchen, but she couldn't help it. Jake had his appointment this afternoon and she could hardly wait for him to get home. She knew it could take up to a week or longer for the lab to process the sample and Dr. Moyer to call them with results, but she still wanted to hear how it had gone. She had prayed near constantly the entire time he'd been there and he should be on his way home by now.

She felt badly for him having to go through this. She couldn't imagine how awful it must have been for him to have to do something like that. And around other people no less! She'd heard that often the rooms were not far from the waiting area.

She also felt partially responsible. Like if she was normal and could have given him a baby by now, he wouldn't have had to go through this. She knew that it was in the Lord's hands and she shouldn't think that way, but sometimes she couldn't help it.

She wandered into the living room and sat on the couch and turned the TV on and began flicking through the channels to try to distract herself. She heard a car door and practically jumped up off the couch and rushed around the corner and into the entryway to open the door for him. He was walking the short distance from his car to the small four feet by four feet porch they had with a few steps leading up to the door. He must have seen how anxious she'd been because he offered a reassuring smile. She exhaled and willed herself to relax and smiled back. By this time he was up the steps and she stepped out onto the porch and hugged him. "I'm sorry."

He wrinkled his brow and said into her shoulder, "For what?"

She snuggled her face deeper into his shoulder and said, "That you had to go through that. I've had tests too. They are not fun and I'm just sorry you had to."

He was touched by his wife's compassion. He pulled her back and smiled at her again. "Let's get inside."

They went in and sat on the couch and Amy turned the TV down and faced him, obviously ready to hear all about it. He told her everything and watched her face react with compassion a few times, but mainly she just listened intently.

He sighed and leaned back and put his arms above his head. "I'm just so relieved that's over with."

She placed her hand on his arm. "I'm glad it's behind you too." She sighed lightly and added, "Maybe in a week we'll have one answer anyways."

He tried to not look nervous and smiled at her. But he was nervous. Afraid something might be wrong with him and then what? He knew from what Amy had told him she'd learned on her group and from talking to Dr. Moyer that low sperm count was not the easiest to treat. He voiced these feelings to Amy.

She leaned in and hugged him again for a long time. "Good news or bad, we'll get through this. At least this part is simple. One test and we'll know one way or the other. Now if we can just figure out what's going on with me." His heart clenched in pain for a moment. She was right. At least he'd only had to do one test and then they'd know. With her, it wasn't so easy. He knew she wasn't downplaying what he'd been through, just stating the facts that it may take awhile to figure out what was going on with her.

He rubbed her back gently as they still held onto each other. "We'll figure it out, Amy. We've got Dr. Moyer helping us now and we're on the road to answers . . . finally. And God is with us. We should know something soon." He felt her relax some against him and he knew his words had comforted her. He told himself these things all the time. When the weight of it all felt as though it could crush him. It did feel encouraging to be doing these appointments in a way. Because for the past two years it had been nothing but doubt and questions. Hopefully soon the fog would be lifted and they could finally see what was really in front of them and which way to turn. They'd finally have what they'd needed for months and months on end and something that had seemed to evade them for so long.

Answers.

J adie could hardly wait! She and Amy had been e-mailing nearly every day for two weeks and tonight they were meeting up on AOL Instant Messenger to chat. They had continued to deepen their almost instant bond and were quickly becoming good friends. She signed in and waited for the familiar sound effect to signal that someone had signed in: the sound of a door opening. She felt nearly giddy as she waited for her new friend to get online.

She played Solitaire while she waited, but it only took a few minutes for Amy to get on. Jadie heard the door sound and looked at the little AOL module on her screen and saw Amy's username appear: "awhitley77." She double clicked her name to bring up a box on her screen that she and Amy would talk in. The top half showed their conversation, the bottom half was a text box for her to type into, and across the middle was a small toolbar like in Microsoft Word so you could add smiley faces, bold or italicize your text, and so on.

Jadie typed "Hello there!" and hit the enter key to send it. It showed up after her username in the top half of the small window.

"Hey, sorry I'm late!" Amy responded. "Jake got home from work a little late and I just cleaned up the kitchen after dinner."

"No problem!" Jadie typed in.

She was sitting at the computer desk in she and Chase's bedroom and heard him chuckle above the sound of the TV in their living room. She quickly walked to the doorway and glanced at her husband all lounged on the couch with the remote in his hand. She forced a scowl to her face, although she could tell it looked playful. "What're you laughing at, mister?"

He glanced at her and grinned before returning his attention to the TV. "Oh nothing. I could just tell how excited you were to talk to Amy."

"How on earth do you think you knew that?" she said as incredulously as she could manage and placed her hands on her hips.

He laughed again. "Oh no reason, honey. It's just that the chair in there is a little squeaky and I could tell you were fidgeting. Then when I heard her get on I could tell you nearly jumped."

Jadie's cheeks reddened slightly. Her husband could read her feelings even in the next room. "Well, so what if I was excited?" she said, still trying to sound mean.

"Nothing wrong with it. I just think it's cute, that's all."

"Why do you always think everything I do is cute?" she asked as she walked over and grabbed the pillow next to him and gave a playful whack to his arm.

The mischievous grin he was known for filled his face again and his eyes danced. "What's wrong with thinking my wife's cute?"

She smiled and whacked him with the pillow again. "Nothing I guess. I can see I'm not going to get anywhere by trying to talk to you."

He laughed lightly again and she returned to the computer, still smiling.

Amy had written, "So how are you tonight?"

Jadie responded that she was well and asked Amy what they'd had for supper.

After a few minutes of small talk, Jadie remembered something she'd wanted to tell Amy.

jadieann80   Oh! I almost forgot to tell you! I added those pictures of Chase and I to the photo album on the group. I kind of followed your example and did a wedding photo and an every day one.

awhitley77   Oh good! Hold on, I'm gonna open another tab and take a look.

jadieann80   Ok.

Amy was excited to see what her friend looked like. She seemed so sweet and Amy wondered if Jadie looked the way she'd imagined her. She waited a moment for the group's photo page to load and then looked for Jadie's folder. She clicked it and it took only a moment for the pictures to load. She clicked on each of them to make them larger on her screen. She smiled. Jadie was even prettier than she'd imagined. From the wedding picture, she could tell she was a bit shorter and had a petite frame. She had medium brown hair that was pretty long and the most beautiful green eyes. She had a somewhat small nose and her face got narrower as it headed towards her chin. She had splashes of freckles on her nose that spread out onto her cheeks some. She was very cute, but lovely at the same time. Next Amy studied Chase a bit. He seemed to be about medium height and was somewhat medium build; not as broad as her Jake. He had shorter dark blonde hair cut all one length and light brown eyes. He had a great big smile and a very pretty one at that. She could tell from the pictures that he was much like Jadie described him. Happy-go-lucky and charismatic, but also laid back. His mischievous grin reminded her of a cat that had just caught a mouse and his eyes practically sparkled right through her computer screen. It was obvious they adored one another.

awhitley77   I LOVE them Jadie. You are even prettier than I imagined and you and Chase look so happy together.

jadieann80   Awww. Thank you, Amy. :) . . . Did you happen to notice what a shorty I am? :P

awhitley77   LOL. I noticed you were shorter, but I wouldn't say shorty. :)

jadieann80   HAHA! Well, thanks. :) I am only about 5 feet. How tall are you?

awhitley77   I'm about 5'5" or so. Jake is around 6 feet though.

jadieann80   Jeesh! Chase is about 5'8". We'd look like dwarfs next to you guys!

awhitley77   LOL! Hardly.

jadieann80   I hope I'm not prying, but would you mind telling me about your family?

awhitley77   You're not prying at all! I'd love to tell you about them. Let's see, my parent's names are Robert and Ann and I have two sisters: Laura who is married to Paul and Alexandra who is engaged to Thomas. Laura and Paul have a daughter named Suzie, my sweet little niece! Jake has two younger brothers: William and Zack. His mother's name is Victoria and his step-dad is Frank.

jadieann80   How wonderful you have so much family! Do they all live near you?

awhitley77   Umm . . . everyone is within 45 minutes of each other at the farthest and some of us are only about 10 minutes apart. So not bad at all!

jadieann80   Oh, that's great! My middle name is Ann. :) In case you didn't notice from my username. How old is your niece?

awhitley77   She is two. :) And I did notice. ;)

jadieann80   Aww, such a fun age!

awhitley77   So, how about your family? And are they all nearby?

jadieann80   My brother is a Senior in high school and his name is Haden. My parents are Dean and Keira. Chase has an older brother, Finn. He's married to Sarah and my nephew, Charlie, is also two. :) He also has a younger sister, Gracie who is the same age and goes to the same school as my brother. His parent's names are Emily and David. Umm . . . yes, we're all close together. We live about 10 minutes from my family and his family is all within a half an hour or so.

awhitley77   That's great!

jadieann80   I noticed you mentioned your in-laws right off when I asked about your family. Are you close to them?

awhitley77   Absolutely! I consider them my family as much as my own. Obviously it's different b/c I haven't known them as long, LOL, but you know what I mean!

jadieann80   Yes, I do know what you mean. :) I feel the exact same way about Chase's family. It's nice to have so much close family around!

awhitley77   It is indeed!

After talking some more about general things, Amy suddenly wrote:

awhitley77   Wow! I don't know how I forgot about this until now! We got the results from Jake's sperm analysis this morning. The lab took just a little longer than usual. I guess they have been quite busy lately. Anyways ... it wasn't terrible news, but not great either.

jadieann80   Uh oh! What'd they say?

awhitley77   Well, the test checks for quantity, motility (how they move), and morphology (how they are shaped, basically)–among other things. His sperm count was down some. About 20 million and "normal" is 40 million. Although they told us this isn't too terrible. The motility was fine, but the morphology was a bit off as well. "Normal" is for 70% of the sperm to have a normal structure and for Jake it was about 55%. They told us all of this wasn't that bad and could be a lot worse. But it doesn't help our chances either and actually decreases them some, I'm sure, although they wouldn't come right out and say that over the phone.

jadieann80   I'm glad it wasn't worse, but I'm so sorry for the negative news. :(Is there anything they can do to help?

awhitley77   From what I've heard, sperm issues can be difficult or complicated to treat. We'll talk more about options the next time we see our infertility specialist.

jadieann80   Wow, I'm sorry! I will keep praying for you guys.

awhitley77   Thanks. I appreciate it! I don't know though, I did some research and the percentages of what is "normal" can vary. So who knows?

jadieann80   Well, hopefully that won't end up being a hindrance to you guys then. How is Jake doing with the news? I know you'd said he was nervous about it.

awhitley77   He is doing ok. He feels guilty b/c he may be responsible at least partially for our problems. I have a feeling it's more me though. Either way, it doesn't matter. What we both want is a baby and it's not our "fault" if something is wrong.

jadieann80   Aww. I know what you mean. You're right that it's not your fault.

awhitley77   Thanks. It's nice having the group to vent to and now I have you as well. :)

jadieann80   I feel the same way! :)

After a time, they got around to talking about some of the tests Amy had been through.

awhitley77   The first test I had done has a really long name, but is most commonly known as HSG. You get a dye inserted into your tubes and you have an X-ray done to see if they are blocked. This was pretty uncomfortable. I took Tylenol first like the girls on the group suggested but it still hurt some. My tubes didn't have any blockage, thank goodness!

jadieann80   That's good!

awhitley77   Yes, it was! Another test I had done was an Endometrial Biopsy. They basically put a little cylinder inside your cervix to get a sample of your endometrial lining. That too was quite painful. Otherwise I've just had lots of blood tests done at different points in my cycles to check hormone levels.

jadieann80   Wow! I'm so sorry you have had to go through all that! :(

awhitley77   Thanks Jadie. I appreciate your sympathy. Hopefully it'll all be worth it in the end. :)

jadieann80   Yes, I'm sure they'll figure out something soon!

The girls talked a bit more and then signed off for the night. Jadie's heart felt heavy for her new friend. She'd learned so much about infertility in the time she'd been a part of the group and from talking to Amy. She shuddered slightly. She hoped it was something she and Chase would never have to face. She walked into the living room to see poor Chase had passed out some time ago with the TV still on. She smiled and walked over to him and watched him sleep for a moment. He looked so peaceful that she didn't really want to disturb him, but she knew he'd sleep so much better in their bed. She gently shook him awake.

He came to with a start. "Huh? What?"

Jadie laughed.

He rubbed his eyes for a moment and said, "How was your talk with Amy?"

"I'll tell you tomorrow, honey. You need to get to bed. The alarm will be going off before you know it."

He stood slowly and rolled his eyes. "Don't I know it! Alright, as long as you promise to fill me in tomorrow."

She put her arm around his waist and they started walking toward their room. "I promise."

❤ ❤ ❤

Haden Carter hurried to his locker with his History book and notebook tucked securely under his arm. He absent mindedly did the combination on his locker until he heard the familiar click. After he'd placed his books neatly in his locker, he breathed in deeply through his nose and looked fondly around the high school hallways. He tried to soak in the sound of sneakers and flip flops smacking and skidding on the tile floor, the chatter and laughter of his fellow students as it echoed through the halls, and the slamming and opening of lockers all around him. He was a Senior at Providence Christian School. It had opened when he was going into fourth grade and his parents had switched him from homeschooling to the new large school that was only about twenty minutes from his home. He had made friends that first day and for the most part, really enjoyed school. He especially loved when he'd moved to Junior High and High School and he could play sports. He'd dabbled in just about everything, but enjoyed Cross Country and Soccer the best. So for the past two years, those were the sports he'd stuck to so he still had adequate time for his studies. While he was excited and ready to move on with his life, he also knew he would miss being here in a way.

There was one thing, person actually, though that held him back from being extremely excited to be leaving his school. Her name was Gracie Taylor.

He sighed fondly just picturing her. He could still remember Mrs. D, as they'd called her, assigning himself and Gracie as reading partners on his first day of Fourth Grade. He could still remember exactly the way she'd looked then in her jeans and light sweater, her shiny and pretty dark blonde hair that was nearly to her waist, and her beautiful bluish-green eyes looking at him. She had smiled and had the slightest little dimples that had completed her perfection. While he wasn't necessarily interested romantically in girls at that age, he was still taken aback by how drawn he'd felt to her and how he couldn't stop staring at her for some reason. *She's quite pretty ... for a girl who still probably has cooties*, he remembered thinking with a smile. They had been friends ever since. Not super close, but not just acquaintances either.

As he pulled out the books for his next class he could almost sense her presence, like he'd always been able to do, and glanced to his right. Sure enough, there she was. Sweet Gracie. She had just rounded the corner and was heading to her locker which was on the opposite side of the hallway and a little distance from his. She was holding her books to her chest with both arms wrapped around them. She had grown more and more beautiful with age. She still looked strikingly similar to how she had as a young girl, only older and more lovely now. She had always been mature and in his opinion, was everything a young lady ought to be. Kind, modest, serious when she ought to be, dedicated, loyal, fun to be around, and she loved the Lord and lived for Him each day. Sometimes when he'd talk to her, her innocent yet piercing gaze was enough to make his jaw go slack and render him speechless. It could be so difficult for him to stay focused long enough to talk to her at times.

He'd never confessed his feelings for her to any one, and especially not to her! He was shy in a way and he just couldn't for the life of him bring himself to ask her out. It just seemed like it would be awkward and forced. And what if she didn't feel the same way? There was no way on earth he could chance ruining their friendship. There was only one thing worse than watching her from afar and just being friends: her being out of his life completely.

She was smiling now and gently laughed as she talked to one of her friends. The sound gently floated to his ears and he felt nearly lightheaded and someone could have easily knocked him over with a feather at that moment. He could barely watch her from a distance without passing out. He forced his eyes back to his locker as he stuffed some of his books and other things he'd need for his homework tonight into his red backpack. He was just getting ready to head to his last class of the day. He clenched his teeth. *Get a grip, Carter*, he told himself. Sometimes when thinking, he'd refer to himself as "Carter" since that's what his coaches always called him. And it seemed fitting if he was being stern with himself and wanting to exercise some self discipline that he would call himself what they did on the field or in practice. If he couldn't even observe her, how on earth would he ever ask her out? It took everything in him to not look like a crazy person who'd lost his mind to just carry on a regular conversation with her.

But he could almost hear a clock ticking away precious seconds in his head. Soon they'd be graduated and then what? He would rarely see her. The one thing he had going for him was that she was his brother-in-law Chase's little sister. So at least they had some connection. But his side of the family didn't have a lot of gatherings where Chase's family was also present. So the chances of him seeing her were slim. If he didn't make a move soon . . . He sighed and tried to force his mind to other things. *Impossible these days it seems*, he thought. It also intimidated him a bit that she was Chase's younger sister. He smiled just at the thought of his brother-in-law. He was a great guy and a lot of fun to be around and Haden did think of him like his own brother. But that was just the problem. Chase was, understandably, protective of his little sister. And what if he and Gracie did date and things didn't work out? Would it make things awkward with him and Chase? Possibly even with Jadie? He sighed again. It was a tricky situation, that was for sure.

While he had met Gracie in Fourth grade, his sister had also coincidentally met Chase that same year. She was a Sophomore in high school and had gone to Chase's parent's house for a youth group gathering. Three different area church's youth groups got together that evening for a cook out over the fire of hot dogs and s'mores at Emily and David Taylor's house, so both Chase and Jadie were present. Chase was a Junior at the time. After many of the kids had left, just a handful remained; Jadie among them. She'd went into the house and visited for a long time with

Chase, his parents, his brother Finn, and some of the other kids that were still there. Haden would never forget the unmistakable glowing of her eyes when she came home that evening. Jadie had told his mother, who was rapt with her attention on her, all about the Taylor's and especially about a boy she'd met named Chase. She found him mature and grounded and as she'd said at the time "refreshing" compared to a lot of the other boys his age that she knew. Haden had quickly tired of the conversation and the googly-eyed look on his big sister's face and headed to his room. But now he understood his sister's draw to him. He imagined it must be much like the one he felt for Gracie. His sister and Chase ended up becoming friends and started dating Jadie's Junior year and were married when she had just turned twenty-two.

The loud ringing of the bell startled Haden out of his musings. He jumped and looked quickly around to see that all but one or two other students still lingered in the hallway. He slammed his locker shut and jogged towards his next class. *Tardy! Hardly the way to finish out the year*, he chided himself.

If he was going to get good grades for the rest of the year and focus on his finals that were speedily coming towards him, he was going to have to try to think less about Gracie Taylor. Something he felt was nearly impossible. Because he knew deep down how far his affection went for her. Something he only admitted to himself.

Haden was in love with Gracie.

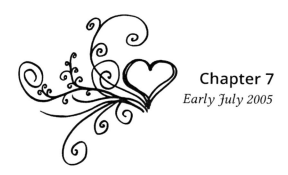

Chapter 7
Early July 2005

Ann Hayes stared into her coffee cup and tried to allow the warmth from it to permeate her cold hands which were both wrapped around her mug, but nothing seemed able to warm her inside. Something was not right with Amy and she knew it as sure as she knew her own name. Something was troubling her daughter, deeply, from what she could see but Amy had not opened up to her and she would not push the matter. Amy had always been more like her father in that way; more quiet and reserved and she didn't open her heart except for those closest to her and only when she was ready. While Ann knew herself to be capable of the same things, she was not quite as reserved as her husband and oldest daughter. And especially as she grew older she had softened some in those areas.

Ann was vaguely aware of her husband moving about the kitchen that was open and connected to the dining room where she sat at the table. She lifted her cup to her lips and took a small sip of her freshly brewed coffee and enjoyed the warm sensation as it trickled down her throat, but it still did nothing to comfort the uneasiness inside of her. She sat her cup back down gingerly and finally registered the fact that her husband had cleared his throat for the third time now. The first two had sounded quiet and distant, but the third one she heard and realized he'd made it deliberately loud to gain her attention. She shook her head slightly and looked to her right. "I'm sorry, Robert." she said sincerely. He was standing on the other side of the counter with his hands palms down on the counter top looking at her intently. "It only now just registered that you were trying to get my attention." He smiled slightly and walked around the counter and pulled out a chair at their table and sat facing her.

"What is it, Ann? You look worried." He was concerned for his wife, but knew it couldn't be anything too serious. They shared everything with each other these days. When they were first married he tended to follow his father's example and not talk to Ann as much about his feelings or ask her about her's, but as the years had gone by they'd realized that their communication–about everything–was vital to their relationship and it was something they'd improved so much over the years. For the past several years now they'd been happier and closer than ever and they always talked about everything.

She sighed slightly and said, "It's Amy. Something is wrong there, I just know it!"

He thought for a moment. "You mean with her and Jake?"

"I'm not sure. I don't think so. They seem connected and strong, but . . . I can't put my finger on it. She's hurting about something; I just don't know what it is." She had turned sideways in her chair and continued to sip on her coffee. She stared into their kitchen and seemed deep in thought.

Robert thought for a moment. If it wasn't Amy and Jake, what else could it be? He too had noticed a slight change in his daughter, especially over the past several months, but he hadn't given it a lot of thought until now. She seemed happy enough at her job at the library. She got along pretty well with her friends from church and she and her sisters rarely got into even mild disagreements.

"Do you ever wonder . . ." he let the sentence hang.

Ann turned to face him again. "What is it, Robert? What are you thinking?"

He looked down for a moment. "It's silly really. I mean I have no idea where to even begin to guess, but . . ."

She was watching him intently now. Her voice and expression were kind and encouraging as she said, "Go on."

"Well, they have been married for over four years now. I knew they weren't in a rush to start a family, but I didn't think they'd wait quite this long either. Maybe it's because of Jake's training and his taking classes? But it just seems like a long time to wait to me. You know Amy was born to be a mother. Don't you remember her fussing over her sisters when they were little?"

"Yes, I do remember. So you're saying . . . you think maybe they're having trouble starting a family?" her forehead was creased with concern.

Robert shrugged slightly. "I don't know. It's possible I guess."

If Ann was honest with herself, she had considered this possibility before. But she'd had no trouble getting pregnant with her girls. She and Robert had only been married a year when they decided to leave things in the Lord's hands and they'd never worried about using protection again until after their youngest, Alexandra, was born. Ann had found out she was pregnant with Amy just a few months after their decision and after each of the girls it took only a year or less before she'd discover she was pregnant again. She and Robert didn't give it a lot of thought at the time. They just figured they were in their child bearing years and they left it up to the Lord. But infertility ran in families . . . didn't it? She couldn't remember where she'd heard that now or if it was from a reliable source. She raised her still hot coffee mug to her face again and breathed in deeply and allowed the steam to caress her face. But it didn't sooth the worry in her. Strange how she felt so chilled today. She pulled her bathrobe tighter around her and stared out at the sunny early July morning.

She glanced at Robert to see he was still watching her, waiting to see if she'd say something. She sighed slightly and said, "I'm afraid you may be right Robert. Amy has always wanted children and even with all they have going on, I still thought they'd at least be expecting by now. I just see the wistful way she watches children at church sometimes and . . ." suddenly she felt her throat tighten and she couldn't finish. The tears coming on had surprised even her. But she'd always loved being a mother and the thought of her daughter aching for that and not having it? It broke her heart.

Robert watched his wife, his eyes filled with compassion for her pain and the pain Amy might be feeling. He covered her hand with his own. "I know, dear, I know." He waited until she'd had a moment to compose herself and when her eyes were no longer brimming with tears he said, "I think that we should just wait for Amy to talk to us like she always has. But worrying won't help us or Amy and Jake. We just need to start praying for her . . . That God would give her a baby in His timing." Ann nodded. He had a strong feeling come over him and he knew the Lord was encouraging them to do just that. The feeling was so strong that he placed his other hand over Ann's and said, "I think we should pray right now."

As her husband began to pray for Amy, Ann closed her eyes and prayed along with her husband. She was a bit surprised how emotional she felt over this. But if Robert's desire to pray right away was any indication, they were both feeling the same way. An urgency that their daughter was going through something and they would help the only way they could right now.

They would pray.

❤ ❤ ❤

Jadie sat at her computer as she often did when she had some spare time. She read through some of her TTC group e-mails. While she and Chase had talked and decided that worrying over when they were going to have a baby was not going to do them any good, she still was so interested in the topic and it was still at the forefront of her thoughts most of the time. She was trying to worry less and pray more these days. She often remembered the song written by John W. Peterson she'd sung in Sunday School as a girl.

Why worry when you can pray?
Trust Jesus; He'll be your stay.
Don't be a "doubting Thomas"
Rest fully on His promise.
Why worry, worry, worry, worry
When you can pray?

She smiled to herself remembering all the times she had sung it with her friends and teachers. But just because she was working on worrying less didn't mean she thought about it any less.

So here she sat, reading the e-mails from her group—one of her favorite things to do. She had already learned so much from these women. Listening to their struggles and seeing all that some of them had been through broke her heart. She knew how badly she wanted a baby and how hard it could be at times for her already and she and Chase had only been trying for about eight months. Some of the women on her group had been trying for a decade. Jadie could hardly imagine waiting that long and how incredibly painful it must be. As she pondered these things, she decided that people were not normally patient creatures so waiting for something like a child when you so desperately wanted one could create not only anxiety, but a deep pain at the thought that it may never happen. Since only God could see the future, a couple really had no way of knowing when things weren't working whether they would ever have children or not. Jadie decided that not being able to see the future and being left wondering over it was just as painful as having to wait to see what would happen.

Amy popped into her mind just then and before she could forget, she closed her eyes and folded her hands in her lap right then and there and prayed for her friend, the women on her group, and anyone else who may be struggling through infertility. She also asked God that He would give she and Chase a baby in His perfect timing, whenever that may be, and that she and Chase would be patient in the meantime. When she was finished praying, she decided to go the bathroom counter to check her latest test.

She and Chase had decided to start using Ovulation Predictor Kits, or as they were known on her group, "OPK'S." Before joining her TTC Group, Jadie had never heard of such a thing or known it even existed. The women on her group had shared that they were much like home pregnancy tests, only they tested to see when you were going to ovulate instead. Jadie had talked it over with Chase and they had decided since they'd been trying for a decent amount of time with no result yet, that it wouldn't hurt to have a better idea of when she ovulated. So about a week and a half ago Jadie had anxiously purchased her first box. It contained twenty-one strips. She had bought the biggest box they had since she wasn't sure when in her cycle to begin testing. She knew about the common belief that most women who had regular cycles ovulated somewhere near the middle of the cycle, around day fourteen. But much to Jadie's dismay, she had learned since joining her group that she'd been keeping track of her cycles wrong. She always wrote down when she started her period, and after about three to four months of TTC she had begun counting days so that they had a rough estimate of when she ovulated. But she had been counting cycle day one as the day after her period had ended. When she joined the group, she realized that cycle day one was the first day of her period. So she had gone back in her notes and used a calendar to get the correct days for all the cycles thus far. So in the months since she had been keeping track they hadn't actually timed their lovemaking as well as they thought they had at times. She had been frustrated over this for a few days, but decided to just be grateful that she knew how to keep track correctly now and that the OPK's would just further help pinpoint the correct time. Jadie was excited about this next step and was sure this would help them have a baby on the way in no time.

When she reached the counter she glanced at the test and the directions which she had lying next to it. Another negative. She couldn't help but sigh. She had been taking the tests for six days now and still no positive. *Can I not even get a positive*

OPK? she thought to herself in frustration. She felt anger and fear building up inside of her and tried to push it back down. She had heard of women on the group that OPK's didn't work for. She couldn't help but wonder if they weren't going to work for her, thus providing no insight or help to her at all. It would also not get her any closer to having something tangible to help her get her baby any time soon. *It's only been six days* she tried to reassure herself. Still, the instructions had a chart and based on how long the cycle normally was they could suggest the day you should begin testing. So she had, but it was six days in and still no positive. She was already on cycle day seventeen. From her group and reading the instructions thoroughly she'd learned that the test picked up the "LH surge" which happened about twenty-four hours before ovulation. So if she hadn't even gotten a positive yet ... It just didn't seem right. She sighed again and then attempted to once again force away the frustration she was feeling. She just assumed that since her cycles had always been regular that she ovulated just fine. *Am I not ovulating? Could that be the problem?* she couldn't help but wonder. But she resolved to not be negative. *It'll be positive soon* she assured herself. She prayed again that God would help her mind not to wander, but to deal with things as they came. She didn't know anything yet, so she should just keep testing until she knew something for sure. If she took them for a few months and never got a positive, maybe she'd see her doctor about it. After she had turned her concerns to the Lord in prayer, a familiar verse came to mind. "So do not worry about tomorrow; for tomorrow will care for itself. Each day has enough trouble of its own." She wanted to write that down so that she could use it in the days ahead if she felt tempted to start worrying over something she didn't even know for sure yet. She headed back to her computer to look up the verse. She typed it in and waited for the verse and reference to pop up. *Ahh, Matthew 6:34. I thought it was in one of the gospels.* She wrote the verse down on a sticky note and stuck it to her computer monitor. She suddenly felt lighter and smiled. *Thank you Lord, for reminding me of that. Help me to not worry and trust in You.* She decided to e-mail Amy an update about the OPK's and the verse that came to her. Maybe it would be of some encouragement to her as well.

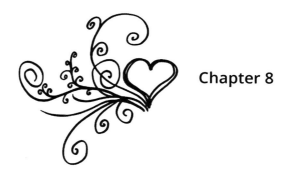

Amy and Jake sat side by side on the examination table at the doctor's office holding hands waiting for Dr. Moyer to enter the room. Most of the time they'd sat in comfortable silence with one another, but occasionally they talked about what this appointment may hold. Sometimes Amy wished with her whole heart that this was just a terrible movie she was watching and not something that was actually happening to her. But as she shifted on the table and heard the familiar crunching sound of the paper and felt her dampened palm against Jake's rough skin, she felt as though all of her senses were heightened and this was very real. This really was happening to her. Sometimes those feelings would come on so strong she felt as though she could not draw breath and would suffocate. What she had faced, what she would continue to face, all the emotion and pain; it just seemed too much at times. She forced herself to breathe normally, said a quick prayer, and was extremely relieved as she felt herself relax.

She turned her face slightly to Jake and gave him a weak, half smile. "Well, she said she had the results of my latest test and that combined with the other things let her know what was going on. I just can't figure out if it's good or bad that she wanted to tell us in person."

Jake felt slightly alarmed at his wife repeating the first part aloud as they'd already talked about it several times. But he reminded himself how nerve-wracking this appointment was and how much was resting on it and assured himself that she was just thinking out loud. As to the second part, he feared it was the latter.

But he squeezed Amy's hand reassuringly and said, "After today, no more wondering."

Amy sighed and visibly even sagged with relief a little.

"Yes, at least that will be nice. Even if it's bad hopefully we can get a game plan and move forward."

Jake smiled just slightly and gave her hand another squeeze.

Amy had another test done since the last time they saw Dr. Moyer. This time they got detailed pictures of Amy's ovaries and uterus. Apparently something that showed up in the pictures must have given Dr. Moyer the answers she was searching for. Soon enough they would receive those answers.

Jake suddenly felt compelled to pray so he turned towards Amy a little and bowed his head. By the time he said the first few words she realized what he was doing and bowed her head as well. His deep voice, although used quietly, resonated in the small room and Amy was both comforted and proud of her husband for thinking to pray.

"Dear heavenly Father, we thank You for all the blessings in our life. We know we have much to be thankful for. At the same time we have a very deep desire to become parents. We know that You know this, Lord, but we ask with all of our hearts that we could get some information today that could lead to us having a baby. Please continue to give Dr. Moyer wisdom as she works with us and help us to accept whatever news we get today in a way that would glorify Your name. Please comfort us as we go through this time, Lord, and give us peace we pray. In Your Son's name, Amen."

Amy felt further relaxed and confident and gave Jake a little smile and squeezed his hand.

Almost immediately after there was a light knock on the door and Dr. Moyer entered. After shaking both of their hands and saying hello as she always did, she sat down and opened their file. She seemed so professional and serious, but also had a warmth about her that both Jake and Amy appreciated. Amy felt her heart may beat out of her chest. All these months of waiting and wondering all led up to this moment. What her Dr. spoke in the next few seconds could and would forever alter her life one way or another. The suspense was about enough to do her in, so she was glad Dr. Moyer got right to the point.

"Amy, after carefully reviewing all of your tests I feel very confident to give you a diagnosis. I am sorry to tell you that you do have Polycystic Ovarian Syndrome."

Amy felt her heart drop to her feet and tried to let the words that were so quickly spoken soak into her and become reality. She and Jake had dreaded this diagnosis and had hoped it wasn't the case. She tried to remind herself that although difficult, it was treatable and she would be grateful for a specific and concise answer and now they could make a plan and follow it.

She steadied herself and waited for the rest. It felt like several minutes had passed when really Dr. Moyer had only paused for a moment.

"I know we had talked about that being a possibility in the past, but I sometimes feel some Doctors diagnose it too quickly and end up being wrong and I wanted to be sure. Your hormone levels were definitely pointing towards it and now that I've carefully reviewed all the results of your tests, especially the most recent one, I feel I can say this with certainty. From speaking to you about this before I know you are familiar with PCOS and what it entails, but I want to go over it with you again. As you know it is caused by complex hormonal complications and causes a woman to not ovulate often or ever on her own. It also can have other ramifications including at some point leading to diabetes."

She continued to pause here and there and try to read Jake and Amy's expressions, but seeing they were soaking it all up, she felt like she could continue.

"I am concerned Amy about some of the tests we've done and I would like you to try to make some changes to your diet that may help get your sugar levels more where I'd like to see them. I have some pamphlets here for you that will help guide you and can also refer you to a dietician if you have more questions or feel it's necessary."

She handed Amy the pamphlets and took in her slightly stunned face.

"I know this isn't the greatest news to hear Amy, but I want to reassure you that this is not your fault and you have not caused this. But now that we know what it is we can help it. I have some information here on Metformin and would like to start you on it right away along with the diet changes to help that issue. I know that this is a lot to take in and that no woman wants to be diagnosed with PCOS as it is complicated and while there are ways to treat it, it often isn't easy. But I feel confident that now that we know what we're facing that we can do our best to conquer it. Do you have any questions so far?"

Amy appreciated her Doctor's straight forward manner, but also starting off with reassurances that Amy desperately needed to hear. Dr. Moyer had leaned forward and been watching Amy intently, but now sat back and waited for Amy to absorb the news and ask questions.

She couldn't think of any, but Jake chimed in with some. Mainly about the side effects of the Metformin and wanting to know how concerned Dr. Moyer was about Amy's sugar levels. Amy felt better after hearing the answers and then thought of something she wanted to ask.

"So I understand about the dietary changes and Metformin to help that part of the PCOS, but what do you feel is the best course of action since I am not ovulating often . . . or ever?"

"Yes, I planned to address that next. While I believe the changes in diet and the Metformin will help your sugar and hormonal levels which could positively affect how your body works including ovulating on it's own, I also would like you to start Clomid to help you ovulate. The changes you make and taking the Metformin will help things over time, but you have already been waiting so long and it's still not a guarantee for ovulation. So I would like you to chart so I can see what your body is doing and take the Clomid and hopefully that will cause you to ovulate well and hopefully achieve pregnancy."

While Amy wasn't thrilled with getting this news, it felt so wonderful to finally see what they were facing instead of stumbling around blindly and have a plan in place to get to their goal.

She shared these thoughts with Dr. Moyer.

"You're right Amy. PCOS is a difficult diagnosis to give or receive, but I am glad that the testing showed us what is happening with your body and we can work on improving things and treating and moving towards what we want to accomplish."

They asked more questions about the medications and taking them together, how the Clomid worked specifically, and how long Amy would be on both meds. Once this was all thoroughly discussed, Jake asked, "What if Amy doesn't get pregnant in the six months on Clomid? Is it safe for her to take it longer or what would you recommend?"

"With patients who have PCOS, I recommend six months of Clomid and should the couple desire further treatment, I suggest then moving to intra-uterine insemination, also known as IUI. If someone with PCOS is not responding properly to the Clomid or is not able to achieve pregnancy within the six months, I feel the best course of action is to move on to IUI." She further explained her reasons for believing that to be the case.

After handing them more pamphlets explaining PCOS and treatment plans and answering a few other quick questions, Amy and Jake shook her hand again and she was gone. Amy felt as though it had all happened in such a blur and was still trying to take it all in. Jake looked worried, but oddly at peace at the same time. He leaned over and hugged Amy who was still seated on the table. "Well, we have an answer and a plan. We are so much further ahead than we were. I am grateful for that. I'd also been worried about you, so I'm glad to know what's going on and how to help. We are going to get through this and come out stronger on the other side. We may still have a journey ahead of us, but at least we're not traveling blindly any more. I'm with you Amy and so is God. We're going to be okay."

Amy couldn't have thought of more perfect words to be spoken to her in that moment even if she would have tried to think of what she wanted him to say. She sagged slightly and wrapped her arms around her husband who was still holding her. A couple of tears slid out of her eyes.

At least we are no longer stumbling blindly Lord. Please be with us. It was a simple prayer, but all Amy could muster for now. God's peace surrounded her and she suddenly felt like she was being held by two sets of arms.

She sighed and a couple of more tears slipped out of her eyes, but this time she was not sad. Everything would be okay.

❤ ❤ ❤

Amy and her family were all gathered at her parent's house and the men had just gone into the living room to watch sports. Amy was hoping an opening like this would come up this evening. It had just been this morning that they'd received her diagnosis at Dr. Moyer's office and in a way it was still sinking in. Jake had given Amy a knowing look that also seemed to say "good luck," followed by a slightly sad smile before he left the room. Since she and Jake could both tend to be rather private people, this was how they'd decided to share the news. Amy would tell her mother and sisters and then allow them to tell the men later. Jake had already called his mother and was allowing her to spread the news to his brothers. She had been very sweet about the whole thing and had sounded sad and told Jake that she and his step-father Frank would be praying.

Amy drew a deep breath and tried to gather her courage as she listened to her sister's chatter about Alexandra's upcoming wedding. Her mother just listened intently and smiled. Amy didn't want to spoil the happy moment, so she forced herself to focus on her sister and joined in the conversation. After nearly forty-five minutes there was a slight lull. It looked as though Laura was just getting ready to say something, but Amy didn't want to wait any longer and figured her sister thought of something else to say about the wedding.

Before she could lose her nerve, she folded her hands on the table and piped up. "There's something I want to share with you all."

Her tone must have been more serious than she hoped because their faces all turned somber and they all three stared at her.

Amy wasn't sure the best way to say it, so she figured she'd just come right out with it. "Jake and I have been trying to have a baby for about two and a half years now." She paused for a moment and watched as shock crossed their faces. "We have been seeing a fertility specialist since March and they've been running tests to determine what is going on. Today we got the diagnosis. I have Polycystic Ovarian Syndrome. It results from a gambit of hormonal issues and can cause a woman to not ovulate on her own often or at all and makes her cycles irregular. It can also cause some other health problems, but we are going to start working on treatment."

She glanced at the faces around her and still saw mostly shock mixed in with some sadness. She waited for a moment and let it all sink in.

Finally her mother turned to her with tears in her eyes. "What? I can't believe this! You've been going through this all this time and all these tests? Why didn't you tell us? We could have at least been praying." Her voice wasn't angry or accusatory, but more like a loud, disbelieving whisper with a hint of hurt laced in.

Amy sighed. This was so hard and she knew she would feel guilt for not sharing this with her family and it only added to all the pain she'd already been through. "It is so hard to explain, mom, where I have been for the past two and a half years. It just felt so private and personal and we just kept figuring it would happen soon. And when it didn't and we started seeing the Doctor, I didn't want to say anything until there was something to tell. I just felt like you all wouldn't understand and maybe I wasn't giving you enough credit and for that I'm sorry. But it was the way Jake and I decided to handle it and it was what I felt was best for us at the time. Do you know what I'm saying?"

Amy had reached out and held her mother's hand while saying this and watched her expression eagerly and waited for her response.

Ann stared at the table for a few seconds and then at her daughter's face. "I understand and am glad you did what you felt was best. I'm just sorry we weren't able to support or pray for you during it. I just . . . I feared this. Your father and I just discussed it recently."

Amy was relieved as her mother spoke and then surprised at the end. "You . . . you did? How did you know?"

"We didn't know. Not for sure. We just knew something was hurting you inside and we figured you'd tell us when you were ready. Things seemed fine with Jake and you and you've been married for quite some time and we . . ."

"You just deduced?"

"I suppose, yes. You were just born to be a mother honey. It was all we could think of that would cause such hurt."

Amy was touched by her mother's words and was surprised a couple of tears filled her eyes. Not one for crying often and especially not in front of people, Amy thought for the millionth time how she seemed to cry a lot lately.

"It's nice to hear you say that, thank you. I just had no idea it was obvious I was hurting."

She glanced at her sisters who had been taking in the conversation so far. They both looked surprised still.

Laura said, "Some things just make more sense now. The way you watch Suzie sometimes . . . there was always such a love there, but . . . but something else too that I just couldn't put my finger on." She had been staring and now looked up at Amy.

"Now I know what I saw. It was longing."

Amy's eyes once again filled with tears at her sister's perception, the way she nailed exactly what was in Amy's eyes when she saw her niece Suzie, and also her sad tone.

She simply nodded.

Alexandra just shook her head in disbelief. "That's just such a long time. I feel so bad you have been waiting that long for something you want so much."

Amy's heart felt as though it would overflow from their simple yet sweet comments. Their compassion was like a balm on her wounded soul.

She squeezed both of her sister's hands and just smiled at them. She forced her tears back where they belonged–away–and then spent the next twenty minutes or so answering questions about her PCOS and the effect it could have on her health.

Amy's heart dropped when her mother asked the next question however. "Dear, do you think that you're just stressing out too much about this? Maybe if you and Jake just relaxed it would happen easier."

Amy breathed in deeply before answering. She had heard women on her group talking about getting told this all the time and how infuriating it was. She did feel frustrated with her mother, but tried to remind herself that her mother knew nothing about this and was just repeating something she'd no doubt heard many times.

"No mom, I'm not stressing too much. To say that this hasn't consumed my thoughts and hurt me deeply would be a lie. But being concerned about a physical problem you have does not cause a problem. People don't get cancer because they are worried about getting cancer, nor did I cause this by stressing that something was wrong. PCOS is a problem with my body that I could not control and did not cause to happen. But now that I know what it is I can work towards helping it."

Amy had said all of this in a very nice tone and also worked at not talking down to her mother. Amy wondered if any one had ever talked to her about this in the past and if so what she had said. She was sure she must have thought much differently and been ignorant to how that all worked before going through it. She wanted to be both respectful of and patient towards her mother.

Ann nodded and said, "Yes, that's true that you have a condition. I just wondered if the stress made it worse is all."

Amy wasn't sure what to say to that and just felt frustration rising again, so she just shrugged.

Alexandra then piped in. "You know, mom and dad said that the Fitzgeralds just adopted a baby. Apparently they'd been trying for like eight years to have a baby of their own and never could and she just found out she's pregnant! Maybe you should just adopt and then it would happen!"

Ann chimed in excitedly, "Yes, that's true! I had forgotten about that." and then smiled at Amy.

Amy had also heard this on her group: that well meaning family members and friends would try to tell you about all these couples they'd heard of adopting babies and then getting pregnant. While Amy didn't think people were making it up, she just felt it was so odd and ignorant that her mother and sister were looking at her expectantly like if she just adopted a baby she would be pregnant. She just stared at them for a few moments, dumbfounded. While she knew both of these things were common responses from people, she was surprised they'd both come out of her family's mouths and in the first conversation she'd ever had with them about this no less.

They just kept staring at her so she finally said, "I don't really even know what to say to that. I'm glad God chose to bless them with a baby through adoption and a biological child and all at once." She worked at keeping her voice even and swallowed and added, "But adopting a baby does not make someone get pregnant. I have a condition and one that I will get treatment for. Hopefully God will allow that to work and give us a baby."

She knew that wasn't a great answer but didn't know what to say.

Her mother said, "Well we know it doesn't make someone get pregnant every time, but it might help. You'd be surprised how many stories I've heard about it!"

Amy just stared at the table and shook her head some. She didn't even begin to know how to make her family understand. Right now she didn't have the energy to try.

Amy listened as they shared more stories of their aunts' cousins' friends' niece who adopted and then got pregnant after years of trying until she wasn't sure she could take it any longer. She suddenly felt glad she had kept this private for so long because although she knew they didn't mean to, it made her feel like they were invalidating her pain and all she'd been through and didn't begin to understand her. She wouldn't have wanted to be told to relax or adopt and then she'd magically get pregnant for the past two and a half years. She wasn't sure how to convey this to her mother and sisters, but at least they had the news now. They must have noticed she'd gone quiet because now they assured her they'd be praying and once again said they were sorry she and Jake were going through this along with quick hugs and then moved back to the wedding talk. Amy felt grateful to know they'd be praying and was relieved the conversation was over.

Laura observed Amy quietly as her younger sister and mother flipped through magazines and talked about dresses and decorations. She could see the hurt in her sister's face and felt badly but had no idea what to say. She and Paul had not struggled to conceive and it was hard to imagine. She was sure it would be hard, but she knew she couldn't begin to understand how hard unless she'd been there herself. Underneath the table she gently caressed the tiny bulge that had appeared on her stomach. She had been about to announce that she and Paul were expecting baby number two when her sister had shared her sad news. Now she was infinitely grateful that Amy had went first. She would keep her news quiet for a bit longer. But she suddenly wondered what it would have been like to still be waiting for this baby to be on the way and not knowing when it would be. She had taken being able to get pregnant easily and start her family for granted. As she watched her sister and could still clearly see the pain in her eyes, she realized she would not do that again. *Thank you God for my sweet baby girl and this precious baby on the way* she prayed spontaneously. *Help me to always remember what a blessing they are from You. And please Lord, let Amy and Jake have a family too.*

Chapter 9

Kendra Atkins drummed her manicured finger-nails on her desk top at the office she worked at over and over again. She stared unblinking at her computer monitor. She shifted in her seat and moved her mouse in little circles to keep her screen from going to sleep as it had already done multiple times so far today. She took a deep breath and let it out slowly through pursed lips and straightened in her seat. She just couldn't focus. Not being able to have a baby was eating her alive. She and her husband, Daniel, had been trying for three years to have a baby. They'd had countless tests and had finally gotten the dreaded diagnosis: unexplained infertility. Even with all the technology there was nowadays, nothing could give them answers and no one could help them. They had been to three specialists and they'd all said the same thing: they didn't know what was going on or why it wasn't working. They had even done a very uncomfortable test where they went to a hotel near the hospital and made love and then went for a post-coital test. Eventually, she and Daniel had decided to pursue IUI, but they did several cycles and nothing ever came of it.

She slid open her desk drawer quietly and looked at the In Vitro Fertilization (also known as IVF) pamphlet lying inside on top of some files. It wasn't break time and she shouldn't be looking

77

at anything personal. She forced herself to close the drawer and anxiously ran her fingers through her hair.

What is wrong with me? She wondered. There were days she swore she was going to have a nervous breakdown.

On the outside she may seem tough and collected, but she was anything but. She was aware that she had insecurities on the inside and had struggled with anxiety often in her life. Only her sweet Daniel was allowed to see what she hid from the rest of the world. He was the only one she'd ever let in and the only one she ever planned to.

Kendra's father had abused her as she grew up and her mother watched it happen. He had ended up in prison when she was in high school and now Kendra had no idea where he was and had no desire to find out. She had since forgiven her mother, but Kendra had resolved early on that she would never be weak like that. Never would she allow someone to control her.

Boys had been interested in Kendra all throughout high school and college, but she paid them no mind. She didn't need a man and would show every one she was completely capable of taking care of herself. Besides, she didn't need love in her life. She was content to be on her own and do as she pleased.

That was until she met Daniel her Senior year of college. She had been having lattes with friends when Daniel walked up with a group of guys. Every one made small talk, but something about him took her breath away. He exuded confidence but didn't have a drop of arrogance. He seemed sweet and somewhat reserved, but also so sure of himself. Most of all his eyes were the most pure and honest she'd ever seen. She tried with everything in her to not be captivated by him, but it was a fight she lost. He later asked a friend for her number without her knowing. He'd called her and against her better judgment she'd talked to him for hours. At the close of the conversation she'd surprised herself a great deal by agreeing to go on a date with him.

A week later she'd met him at a restaurant on a pier in a light, summer dress and they talked and laughed until nearly midnight.

No one had ever made her feel as light and free as Daniel. She always thought she'd feel weighted down by having someone, but he did the opposite. He understood her and he saw straight through to her heart. When she put up walls, he'd torn them right down. He was the only one that could ever do that with her.

She'd found out on that first date that he was enlisted in the military. He was in the Marines and was stationed not too far from her college.

Over time she found herself opening up more and more to him and two years to the day of their first date, they were married. It was a small and simple ceremony, but Kendra couldn't have been more proud to be joined to her soldier, her man, her soul mate. Before meeting him she'd never believed in such things. She never knew any one could love someone so much.

Before Daniel she had not thought of having children much. She thought maybe . . . someday . . . if she ever met the right guy . . . but it was a loose plan and one she was not sure if she'd ever follow since she had been completely happy to be on her own. But Daniel had changed all of that. Suddenly she had pictured them in the future and not just the two of them, but with children. At first the realization startled her, but then it grew on her. He wanted children too and he opened up a part of her heart that she hadn't known existed. By the time they had started trying for a baby she was so ready to be a mother she could taste it. No one was allowed to know the real Kendra, but she resolved that when it came to her family—Daniel and their children—she would be herself and let them in and give them all the love she had to give. What a beautiful picture that painted: she and Daniel . . . a family along with their little ones.

She smiled and then snapped back to the present with a start and schooled her features. She quickly glanced around to see if anyone had seen her staring into space and then smiling like an idiot. It seemed that no one had.

Get a grip, Kendra! Focus! She scolded herself.

She grabbed her purse to head to the ladies room which was

only a few yards from where her desk was. She told herself she would splash some water on her face and clear her mind and would come back out and get some work done. With that resolve in mind, she took off like a woman on a mission to the restrooms.

Emma Simmons watched as her Manager, Kendra, strode to the ladies room with a purpose. Emma's desk was off to the side of Kendra's and she often couldn't help but observe Kendra. Emma noticed that she seemed so in control and poised much of the time. Then other times, when she thought no one was watching, she seemed sad and distracted. Or just a few moments ago Emma had caught her daydreaming and smiling. Something about Kendra made Emma's heart squeeze in pain a lot of the time. She wanted to approach Kendra, but if she was honest with herself, she was terribly intimidated by the woman. She was cold and aloof and although she occasionally offered a smile, even that was professional and the walls were always up in her eyes. As Emma watched the tall, slender women shut the door behind her, she wondered what had caused her to be the way she was today and why she often looked so sad. She had long, jet black hair and dark eyes and was fair skinned and quite striking. She seemed like a woman who could get anything she wanted professional or otherwise. So what was she lacking?

Emma hoped one day she'd be brave enough to find out. And tonight she would ask her husband Steve to pray with her about it.

♥ ♥ ♥

Amy could feel her pulse in her fingers as she held the phone to her ear and anxiously waited. She had to admit to herself that she was a bit nervous about calling Jadie for the first time. They had only e-mailed and talked on instant messenger until now and while Amy felt as though she'd known Jadie for years, it was still a bit nerve wracking to be getting ready to speak to her for the first time. She still marveled often over how fast they had bonded. Amy had never felt as drawn to any one in her life and she knew the Lord had placed Jadie in her life for a reason. She hadn't told Jadie yet, but she'd been such an encouragement and blessing to Amy already. With infertility and also spiritually. It was lovely to have a sister-in-Christ and dear friend all in one sweet package.

She cleared her throat anxiously as the phone rang for the third time. She had made sure that Jadie had the afternoon off from the flower shop so she would be home when she called. Not only did she want to get this first call over with as she had a feeling they would be friends for years to come and would want to talk on the phone, but she also wanted to tell her friend and hear her reaction to her news over the phone which was as close as she could get to talking to Jadie in person. When Amy was just beginning to wonder if Jadie was outside perhaps or somewhere where she couldn't hear the phone, she heard her friend answer in a winded tone. "Hello?"

Amy couldn't help but smile at her friend's sweet and nearly youthful sounding voice. It suited her so well.

"Hello, Jadie. It's Amy."

Jadie's surprise and delight rang through the line and echoed in Amy's ears. "Amy! Hello! It's so wonderful to hear your voice."

"Thank you. You too."

Amy felt suddenly shy and embarrassed that she felt that way. Even though there'd only been the shortest of pauses, Amy felt as though the time drug on forever and the silence was deafening. She scrambled to think of something to say, but Jadie beat her to it.

"Sorry it took me so long to answer! I was outside doing some weeding in the flower beds around the house and forgot to take the cordless outside with me. That's why I sound like I just ran a marathon."

Amy felt herself relax a little and chuckled. "That's okay! I was just hoping you were home."

They chatted for a few minutes until Amy noticed that she suddenly felt completely at ease. She could tell by Jadie's tone that she was more relaxed as well. She forged ahead with what she had to tell her friend.

"So, a big part of the reason I wanted to talk to you was because I wanted to tell you about our appointment the other day with Dr. Moyer."

"Yes! The big appointment. I was trying to keep myself from being rude and asking you right off." She followed this up with a light laugh.

Amy laughed softly for a moment. "Oh it wouldn't have been rude. I'm glad you're anxious to hear about it. Well, we got some not so great news. But at least we know how to proceed from now on."

"Oh, Amy, what is it?" she asked with genuine concern.

Jadie's gentle and sweet nature was nearly too much for Amy and she was surprised she suddenly got choked up by her friend's compassion. She swallowed a couple of times and forced her voice into a normal tone as she continued. "Well, I was diagnosed with PCOS for sure. As you know our Doctor had suspected it for a time, but we were hoping that wasn't the case. Like we've talked about before, PCOS is not something you want to have due to the ovulation trouble and even though it is treatable, it can still be a tough and long journey. It's also kind of scary to know that it could cause me other health problems."

"Oh Amy! I am just so sorry. I know God knows what He's doing, but that doesn't mean it isn't a hard thing to go through. I will pray extra hard. Can you tell me about the other health problems and what the plan of action is?"

Once again Amy was touched by Jadie's sweet nature and went on to explain the answers to both of Jadie's questions just as she had to her mother and sisters.

Amy and Jadie ended up talking for over an hour and when they hung up Amy realized something. While she was touched by her sister's and mother's responses and she appreciated their concern and love for her, it just wasn't the same as talking to someone who at least somewhat knew what she was going through. Alexandra was not married and Amy knew she couldn't even begin to fathom what she and Jake were going through. Amy knew she had never understood what people going through infertility faced. Especially when she was engaged and a newlywed, when the future shone so bright with promise. Laura had absolutely no trouble conceiving Suzie and her mother never had trouble either. While she knew they cared, it was still so difficult to listen to some of their comments. Her mother had even called her again since that evening and told her how important it was that she not be stressing over it because it would just make it harder to conceive. She had also suggested they take a vacation as that had worked for many other couples. Amy knew her mother loved her with her whole heart, but she was so hurt by that and instead of attempting to explain it to her mother, she just shut down and tucked the hurt in her heart. Jadie had only been trying for about nine months, but she already could understand how the waiting and wondering could wear on a person and how awful it was to face the question "will we ever have children?" Never once had Jadie told her to not stress, how if she just relaxed it would magically happen, and so on. She was just compassionate, said she would be praying, or things of that nature. Jadie didn't even need to say much; Amy knew their hearts understood one another and it meant a great deal to her. After speaking with her on the phone she felt even closer to her.

So close in fact that she wondered what she had ever done without her.

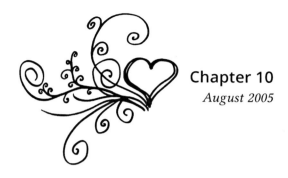

Chapter 10
August 2005

There were tables set up everywhere under two tents and also out in the sun and every one of them seemed to be full of people. Jadie glanced around as she held her plate of food to see if there was somewhere she could sit. She noticed the picnic table by her parents back porch and near some landscaping was vacant so she headed that way. The smell of smoke and meat from the grill wafted through the breeze along with lots of voices and laughter. It was almost surreal to be at her brother's graduation party. It had seemed to come fast and slow all at once. She could hardly believe he had already graduated; it seemed like she was just graduating high school! At the same time, with the age gap between them especially, it did seem like she had been through a lot since graduation including being married to Chase for over three years now. She shook her head. Time was a strange thing indeed.

The graduation ceremony had been lovely. The speakers were great and she loved watching the slideshow of the students of the Senior class as some other students sang a song or two. She watched the tears roll down the faces of many of the students, guys and girls alike, as they reflected on all of their memories together and looked forward to their futures which they would face without each other. It was bittersweet and she remembered

Chapter 10

the feeling well. Although she loosely kept in touch with most of her classmates and had a couple she talked to regularly, it was never the same and the graduation ceremonies always held a bit of finality to them. But mainly she'd just felt very proud and even wiped a couple of tears away as she watched her brother stand tall and handsome in his black cap and gown receiving his diploma. It felt like just yesterday, but really the ceremony had been the first week of June. Two months had passed already!

As she bit into her cheeseburger and thought about how wonderful it tasted, she also reflected on how much time seemed to be on her mind these days. She found herself wishing away the days at times and while she didn't want to be that way, it was hard not to. At the beginning of her cycle she couldn't wait to get further into it so it was close to ovulation time. Then she both dreaded the two week wait until she would find out if this month finally worked and wished it would go slower so she could hold onto hope. Once she always found out it was a no go once again, she looked forward to ovulation time again. She also thought about how much time was passing; time she could be pregnant or have with her child. Yet she was rushing the months to get to the next one so she could try again.

Chase plopped down next to her and she jumped slightly and came out of her musings. "Hey there, gorgeous."

She couldn't help but smile at her husband's tanned face, sparkling eyes, and charming smile.

"Hey yourself. The food is great."

"Oh yeah? I'm starving so I'm sure it'll taste good regardless."

Jadie laughed. She popped a grape in her mouth and once again surveyed her parent's back yard and all the people who had come out to support Haden.

"There sure are a lot of people here!"

Chase groaned and rolled his eyes back as he enjoyed a very large bite of his hamburger.

Jadie once again laughed at her husband.

"Yeah, that's heavenly! Your dad sure knows how to grill. And

86

yeah, there are a ton of people! I asked your dad and at last count he said they'd already had two hundred guests."

"Wow, that's amazing!"

Haden walked up right then with his hands in his pockets. "What's amazing?" He put his finger to his chin and looked up innocently. "Oh wait! You must be talking about me." and then he flashed a grin at them both. Jadie smiled and shook her head. His mischievous little comments reminded her sometimes of Chase.

Chase said in an over-exaggerated tone, "That's right!" and then stood slightly and clasped Haden's hand and then pulled him in for a one armed hug.

Jadie just rolled her eyes and then gave her brother a quick hug. "We were just talking about what a great turn out you have had today!"

Haden responded, "Oh yeah. I was surprised how many people came." Haden allowed his eyes to roam while he talked to his sister and brother-in-law. "I think it's because I did it later in summer since every one . . . well that is, people in my class, they . . . they tended to do their's right after . . . right after . . ."

Jadie got a puzzled expression and followed her brother's gaze to see what had caused his attention to drift so badly. She craned her neck around until she saw Gracie with Chase's parents talking to her mom and dad. She cocked her head slightly and looked at her brother.

Chase quickly figured out what had caught his gaze as well and playfully punched Haden in the arm. "After what? Spit it out, buddy!"

Haden physically jerked and then whipped his head back to them, eyes wide. "Oh . . . uh, sorry. Right." He cleared his throat awkwardly. "They, uh, did their parties right after graduation so it was a busy time. Mom was wise to suggest we do it later in the summer so more people could come. After most people go on vacation and before moving to colleges and such." Once he got that out he gave an awkward laugh and rocked on his heels with his hands in his pockets.

Jadie worked at not smiling. She had sometimes wondered if Haden had a crush on Gracie, but she'd never noticed how much of an impact she had on Haden. But she didn't want to embarrass her brother, so she wouldn't say anything. Especially not now.

Chase took a drink of his Pepsi and then said, "Yeah, that's true. Your mom's one smart cookie."

Jadie wrinkled her brow and said, "You're in fine form today."

He looked at her and winked. "It's a nice and happy day is all. Can't a guy have a little fun?"

She laughed. "Of course you can. You just seem extra . . ."

"Charming . . . amazing . . . dashing . . ."

Jadie laughed again and lightly slapped his arm. "Full of spunk today."

He shrugged and forced a serious tone as he said, "That's one way to put it."

Jadie rolled her eyes and smiled and looked at her brother again. She noticed they'd lost him again however.

"Haden, do you want to go say hi to the Taylor family?"

He was nearly standing on his tip toes now and moving his head slightly back and forth.

Chase glanced at him and cleared his throat loudly. Haden didn't respond so Chase turned and shoved him gently and said in a slightly raised voice, "Hey Carter! What's so interesting over there?"

Haden fell back a bit and caught himself. "Huh? Oh, nothing! Sorry. I . . . uh . . . I think I'm gonna go say hello to your parents."

Chase made his voice sound stern and had hunkered down over his food slightly. "And my sister?"

Jadie looked at him and was surprised at his very serious face and almost piercing gaze.

"Well, yeah, her too." Haden said in a shy and suddenly uncertain tone.

Chase simply made a strange noise by quirking his lip and then went back to eating.

Haden held his hand out and said, "I'll catch you guys later."

"Okay, Haden. See you in a bit."

After she'd called that out to her brother's retreating back she turned to her husband. "What was that all about?"

Chase wiped his face with a napkin. "What?"

She gestured with her hand toward the direction Haden went in. "That! That with Haden. What was that about?"

"Well he's clearly infatuated all of a sudden." He took another bite and swallowed and muttered, "Twitterpated might even be a better word."

Jadie was flabbergasted. Chase loved Haden and even if he thought Haden was interested in Gracie she figured he'd be happy about it.

"So . . . what's wrong with that?"

Chase looked at her and then slowly let one of his most mischievous smiles fill his face. Jadie was truly perplexed by her husband. "Nothing, honey. I just noticed he seems suddenly interested and well . . . she is my sister." He turned back to his food. "I just want to make him sweat a bit."

Jadie's eyes had grown huge. "Chase Taylor! You're terrible! Making poor Haden suffer. He's probably petrified of you."

"Ahhh. It's good for him."

Jadie shook her head once again. "You really are in a mood today!"

Chase merely shrugged and grinned at her.

Haden wiped his sweaty palms up and down quickly against his jeans before reaching the Taylors. He tried to steady his thundering heart, but didn't succeed before reaching them. He shook David and Emily's hands and thanked them for coming and then turned to Gracie. She was wearing khakis and a pastel colored shirt and she looked perfect. Before he could lose his nerve he forced himself to give her a quick hug which she returned and then beamed at him. The hug was enough to make him weak in the knees and now he felt like he'd just been sucker punched and struggled to draw breath. He finally managed to ask how she was and she answered easily. *I wish I could make myself converse with you that easily* he thought. After a few minutes of agonizing small talk, her parents wandered off to say hello to some of the other guests and get something to eat. Gracie started wandering from her place in front of the garage towards the tents in the backyard and Haden easily followed. The small talk had given Haden time to calm down, but he was so nervous and so ready to talk to Gracie alone at the same time. She kept the conversation as easy as her pace and Haden found himself being able to give intelligent responses as long as he looked at his feet and where he was walking.

Finally they stopped in the middle of the yard. They were out of hearing distance of the other guests and she turned to face him again. He sucked in a deep breath as he looked into her piercing gaze again. Those eyes. He was pretty sure God had never created more beautiful eyes in a person than Gracie Taylors'.

She reached out and gently touched his shoulder, concerned. "Are you alright?"

He quickly shifted his shoulder so her hand fell because he had to break contact. This girl had no idea what she did to him when she was near. When she touched him like that it made him want to be an idiot and just blurt out that he loved her more than life itself and take her in his arms and never let go. He couldn't do that obviously, so he shrugged her off and said quickly, "No, I'm fine. I get allergies sometimes in the summer." It wasn't a lie although it wasn't why he couldn't breathe at that moment.

"Oh, okay." She quickly withdrew her hand and looked slightly hurt and then glanced down and did something he recognized she did when she was uncomfortable: she tucked her hair behind her ear several times even though it was in place after the first time.

Haden felt like a jerk, but he couldn't tell her what he was thinking or why he'd shrugged her hand away so fast. *Man, I'm already messing this up so fast!* he thought. He scrambled for something to say to reassure her or be kind to her and bring a smile back to that sweet face. Time was passing and the silence was awkward.

He ducked down slightly and tried to get her to look at him and made himself use a tone that he'd heard Chase and other guys use. A sweet and soft tone.

He simply said, "Hey" and added in his nicest smile.

She shyly glanced up at him and he was surprised as her cheeks went a bit pink. She glanced down again for a moment and then forced her eyes to his.

Keep the conversation going. Say something, Carter! "So. We were talking about school and our friends and I just realized that I'm not sure where you're going to college."

She seemed relieved to have something to talk about again and maybe even that he still wanted to talk to her. He couldn't be sure.

They talked about that for awhile and while neither was set on a college, it sounded like they both wanted to attend a Christian college and one not too far from home.

Secretly Haden hoped with all of his heart that they ended up attending the same school.

He made sure to talk to other guests and eventually he and Gracie got something to eat, but they stayed close the rest of the day. He didn't realize how long they'd been talking but suddenly he saw that the sky was beginning to darken slightly and beautiful colors began splashing along the horizon.

They were standing in the same part of the yard as they had been earlier that day. Gracie crossed her arms and turned towards it and breathed in deep. "It's so beautiful isn't it?"

He looked at the waning sunlight gently caressing her skin and the way it made her eyes an even more remarkable shade and sent soft glimmers through her hair. He allowed his eyes to skim her face several times since she wasn't looking at him. His voice came out a little quiet and hoarse. "Yeah. Very beautiful." He forced his eyes to the sunset.

He wanted so badly to take her hand in his, but he felt it would be inappropriate when she didn't even know how he felt.

He suddenly realized as they watched the sunset together for a few minutes that God created each person and each sunset somewhat the same. They were all different, unique, special, and beautiful in their own way. He realized he'd always remember the beauty of what he was watching now since it fell on the day of his graduation party and also because of the sweet moments he'd gotten to spend with Gracie. But the beauty next to him he wanted to cherish all of his days.

♥ ♥ ♥

Amy had taken her Clomid a couple of weeks ago now. It felt wonderful to finally be doing something that may actually lead to them achieving pregnancy after all this time. She was trying to be hopeful, but also to not have her hopes too high. She realized that her PCOS diagnosis could make this still not work for her or at least not in the six months they had to try. She resisted sighing. Sometimes it seemed that everything was so much harder for them than it was for everyone else. She instantly caught herself and prayed apologizing for thinking that way. That wasn't true and Amy knew it. She and Jake had been very blessed in life; this was just one area they were struggling in. She did sometimes wonder why, but she knew everyone had problems and there were many things in the world that were more horrible than what she was going through. At the same time, if she always compared her struggles to other people's, she could always come up with someone who had worse things going on. Did that mean her problems didn't matter?

Dear Lord, please help me to view this in the right light. This is painful and just because there are worse things in the world doesn't mean my struggle isn't valid. But also help me to not blow it out of proportion or view everything negative. Thank you for all You have given us. I pray that You would help us through this time and please help the medicine to work. Amen.

Amy had learned as a person, and especially as a Christian, that her mind was a battle ground. She had been working hard lately at jumping on negative thoughts that seemed small, insignificant, or that she would normally "let slide," right away instead of letting them fester and grow.

She tried to focus on how positive it was that she was now being treated for her problems and problems that were no longer gray areas, but that had been clearly identified. Those things in themselves were huge blessings.

Amy had already known quite a bit about Clomid before her Dr. ever prescribed it. From the group and what little research she had done on infertility, she knew it was probably the most common medicine prescribed in the infertility world. She had read somewhere once that approximately a quarter of all female infertility issues stemmed from ovulation problems. Clomid was the most common treatment for it. Some women on the group had experienced nausea, hot flashes, mood swings, or other symptoms while taking it. In most cases they were mild. But some women complained of weight gain and that was a dreaded side effect for any woman. So far Amy hadn't noticed a difference in her weight. In fact, she had lost a couple of pounds now that she knew how to eat better for her condition and she'd also been working on exercising a few days a week. The only thing Amy had experienced was hot flashes and she didn't get them often and they weren't too severe. At this point she was willing to put up with nearly anything if it got her closer to finally having a baby. Still, she felt bad for the women on her group who had a hard time with it or whose symptoms were strong from it. She remembered back to before she and Jake had started trying to have a baby: she never once thought about what people who struggled to get pregnant went through. It just didn't seem that widely talked about or acknowledged in society. Now she understood why. Not only did it feel personal or even shameful so couples kept it to themselves, but oftentimes when someone did share they didn't receive much sympathy or understanding. In fact quite the opposite at times and it only added to the person's isolation and pain. Amy shuddered remembering what some members of her TTC group had shared about things people had said to them. They were things Amy couldn't imagine saying to someone she disliked, let alone a family member or friend. Even if the person saying the cruel things didn't completely understand infertility, she figured they had to be able to figure out that their words would at the least be hurtful. Unfortunately some people were thoughtless. That's when the other girls on the group would rally around the hurt person and defend them, validate them, and encourage them. Amy was grateful every day that she had found that group. Especially since she'd met Jadie. They were growing closer all the time and Amy felt truly blessed to have her new sweet friend.

Sunlight streamed through the windows and Amy smiled as she soaked that in along with the sounds of birds chirping outside. She continued to work on her housework in an attempt to have it all done by the time Jake got home. She continued to marvel that being on Clomid may actually help her ovulate since she hadn't been doing much, if any, of that on her own. Her Dr. had prescribed fifty mg pills which she had taken on cycle days five through nine. That should have caused her to ovulate shortly after and now it was a waiting game to see if anything had happened. Amy didn't have her hopes up too much for this cycle, but it still felt good to know that her body may actually start doing what it should in the next few months. It gave them a chance that they hadn't had before and Amy was grateful.

Somehow the time flew by and all of Amy's chores were done. Jake should be arriving home in about twenty minutes, so she decided to quickly check her e-mail from the group. She also hoped she had another e-mail from Jadie. Jadie had already mentioned a few times that Amy was such an encouragement to her. What Jadie didn't realize was how much good she did for Amy's heart as well.

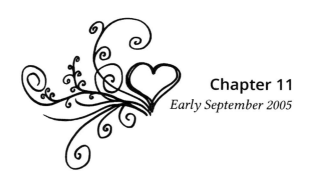

Chapter 11

Early September 2005

Emma stood and took a deep breath, tugged at the ends of her suit jacket and walked purposefully towards Kendra. It was their lunch break and Kendra and a couple other co-workers were standing a little ways off from Kendra's desk but not quite to the break room. Emma had made attempts a few times in the past weeks to approach her, but Kendra was always quick to shut her out and move on to something else. Not to be deterred, Emma strode up and smiled at each woman and finally planted her gaze on Kendra.

"How are you today, Mrs. Atkins?"

Kendra looked slightly surprised and then Emma tried to not visibly jump as the walls clearly just multiplied and fortified in her boss' eyes.

"I am fine, Mrs. Simmons." she replied in a rather brusque tone.

"Please, call me Emma." she gently reminded her and not for the first time. "I'm glad to hear you are well."

Kendra simply continued to stare at her, seemingly surveying her and challenging her to dare continue at the same time.

Emma folded her hands to keep them from trembling and forged ahead. "How are the plans coming for Mr. Davis' surprise party?"

Their employer had a milestone birthday coming up and all

the women in their department had been working on preparing a party.

Kendra didn't have a chance to reply as the other women chimed in with responses of their own. But to Emma's surprise, Kendra stayed and attempted to participate in the conversation. After a few more minutes of small talk, the other women went to their desks to retrieve their lunches and headed to the break room. Before Kendra could dart off as well, although she didn't seem in as much of a hurry as usual, Emma attempted to speak to her directly again. When she couldn't get but a few words out of her in each response, she decided to not push it and let her boss go.

She cleared her throat and forced herself to say, "Well, enjoy your lunch! I will be praying for you."

She turned to walk away but Kendra's voice stopped her. "What did you say?"

Emma turned to face her again and said gently, "I said I will be praying for you."

For the first time she saw Kendra look genuinely puzzled. "Why would you pray for me?" She seemed to catch herself and cleared her throat and glanced down awkwardly. "I mean . . . that is . . . if you don't mind me asking."

Emma was surprised to see any kind of softness from her and didn't mind at all answering her question. She shrugged slightly. "I pray for all my co-workers and you are no exception. I care about you, so I pray for you."

Kendra's look softened a bit more, but then she straightened herself to full height and gave a curt nod. "I see. Well . . . thank you." Then she quickly began to walk away.

Emma smiled inwardly. While she tried to look domineering, the walls had not gone back up in her eyes. *I think I may have just made a little progress* she thought happily to herself.

As she walked towards her desk her happiness quickly flew out the window as a stabbing pain in her middle took her breath away. She quickly leaned over and placed one hand on her desk top to stabilize herself and the other clutched her stomach. She breathed deeply and waited a moment, but a stronger stabbing pain hit her again and she lightly gasped. Kendra's desk was not far from her's and she must have heard Emma's gasp because she came rushing over.

Kendra was all business and talked to her in a calm but nearly stern voice. But for some reason it did not intimidate Emma, but comforted her. She could tell Kendra was not being rude but was genuinely concerned.

"Emma, are you alright?"

When Emma only shrugged she drew closer and gently placed her hand on Emma's shoulder. "Where does it hurt? In your stomach?"

Emma nodded and continued to try to breathe evenly in and out. Right then another sharp pain hit her and she winced and moaned and nearly dropped to her knees.

Kendra gently took Emma's elbow and lowered her onto her chair. "Do I need to call 911?"

Emma's heart pounded so loudly she swore Kendra could probably hear it. Her eyes slid shut in pain that was far deeper than physical as she realized what was happening. *Dear God, please no.*

She'd had a positive pregnancy test about five weeks ago and this was the furthest she'd ever made it into a pregnancy. *God, please don't let this happen again. I can't do it!*

Kendra studied Emma's pale face and watched as tears slipped out of her closed eyelids. Her concern mounted especially since Emma had not answered her last question. She studied her medium height employee with light brown hair that went down past her shoulders. She had light to medium brown eyes, an infectious smile, and while Kendra would never admit it to any one, she found Emma to be rather sweet and something about her drew her in a little although she had tried very hard to fight it off. Just then Emma winced and moaned again and clutched her stomach with both hands and Kendra decided to take matters into her own hands.

She picked up Emma's phone and was about to dial when Emma reached out and grabbed her wrist. "What are you doing?" she asked, wide-eyed and fearful.

Kendra's heart clenched but she tried to ignore it. "I am calling 911. You need help right away. You look like you're about to go into shock."

Emma shook her head vehemently back and forth. "No . . . I'm okay. It just . . . hurts. But I think I know . . . I . . . I just need to get to the bathroom to check something."

Kendra wanted to fight her on it but could tell that Emma would not budge on her position. She had never seen her so serious and set on something.

"Very well. I will help you to the bathroom and wait for you, but if you are still not feeling well I must insist we get you some help. Deal?"

Emma was in too much pain to analyze how her boss spoke to her more gently than she ever had and how kind she was being. "Fine."

Emma tried to not double over as they headed for the bathroom. On top of the occasional stabbing pains, she was having cramping in her stomach and it was spreading to her lower back. For a few moments she had tried to convince herself that maybe this was normal. But she knew in her gut that nothing was right about this. Kendra released her arm when they reached the stall.

Emma tried to fight her tears, but still they made their way down her cheeks as she sat down. *Please God . . . I'm begging you. Don't let it be the baby. Please let the baby be okay.* She and her husband Steve had been through four miscarriages in the last year and a half. This would be number five. It just couldn't be! The answer was probably right in front of her and she knew she had to know.

She shut her eyes and then forced herself to look at the toilet paper in her hand. Her breath caught in her throat and she choked on a sob.

A horrifying dark red blood.

She whispered frantically, "No. No. No. No. No. This can't be happening. This is a dream."

Kendra could hear her whispering outside the stall and gently rapped on the door. "Emma, are you alright? I really think we should call someone now."

Emma wiped at her tears and tried to mentally slow her heart rate down. The way it slammed wildly and so fast in her chest reminded her of the sound of a horse's hooves as it ran full speed. *Yes, I need to get to a hospital. Maybe there is something they can do.*

"Emma . . . I really think . . ."

Emma cut her off. "Yes! Umm . . . yes, can you call my husband? His number is the first one in my contact list on my cell. Top drawer on the left. He can pick me up and take me somewhere."

"I will be right back!" Kendra said with an urgency but also a warning in her tone that made Emma afraid to move from that spot until she got back.

Everything happened in a blur after that and Emma felt as though she was watching everything happen to someone else. Waiting in pain for an agonizing twenty minutes for Steve to arrive with Kendra hovering over her, the ride to the hospital, Steve's wide eyes and frantic questions, being admitted at the local ER and waiting for a Doctor to see her, and finally a blood test followed by an ultrasound. Hearing the horrifying words "no heartbeat" followed by sympathy from the Doctor and an appointment for the next day to have a D&C done, which was the worst part. But even on the ride home she remained dry-eyed and in shock and stared unblinking out the window. She was watching a horror film . . . that was it. There was no way this was happening to her . . . not again.

Back at the office Kendra was nervous and on edge for the rest of the day. She frequently thought back on her co-workers admission that she'd been praying for her. She had felt as though someone had struck her when Emma said those words it surprised her so much. Daniel had just told her about a week earlier that he had accepted Christ as His Savior. She didn't know what to make of this, so she'd asked him for time to process. He'd been very patient with her about it. It didn't bother Kendra as much as she thought it might have that her husband had "found God." Kendra had always believed that something of a Higher Power must exist because she didn't buy for one minute that the Universe and all it contained simply happened. Still, her husband was strong and capable . . . a Marine even! She was surprised he felt a need for God. And it had made him an even more amazing person and the peace he radiated was so tangible and real that it startled her. It gave her a lot to think about. And now Emma saying she was praying for her. Did Emma pray to Daniel's God she wondered? There were many gods and religions she knew. She assumed Emma was probably of the Christian faith as well but she hadn't been brave enough to ask. She shook her head. Actually she realized she'd been too proud to ask. Even asking why Emma was praying for her was letting her guard down and she would not allow the discussion to continue. She found it sweet, touching even, that Emma had admitted that to her. Especially after she'd held her at arm's length.

And now she found herself fretting over her co-worker. As a private person herself Kendra would never ask what was going on with Emma. But she did wish to know if Emma was alright. She was surprised she cared this much, but then, why shouldn't she? She wasn't a monster after all! She did have compassion for people . . . didn't she? She had been pacing but now plopped down in her office chair and slumped. She realized with a sadness that was hard to describe that she often didn't care about others or what happened to them. *Am I that hard and cynical?* she pondered, but then felt the familiar need to sit up straight and a familiar thought raced through her mind. *No. You're just protecting yourself and there's nothing wrong with that.* Kendra suddenly wondered for the first time where those thoughts came from and why she had them. Would she really hold herself away from people her entire life just because she thought her mother should have protected her?

She quickly slid her office chair up to her desk and quickly began working. *Enough thinking for today.* She hoped Emma was alright. In fact she was afraid to admit even to herself she was half tempted to pray for her . . . however one went about doing that. But she didn't want to let her own rambling and confusing thoughts consume her. And she was at work after all. So work she would and put these things from her mind.

♥ ♥ ♥

Amy fanned herself as she looked around at all the other people seated around her. *I'm glad she had such a nice turn out*, she thought to herself. Her sister Alexandra deserved every happiness and Amy wished her much of that today especially as it was her wedding day. All the guests were seated on white plastic chairs in a half-moon shape around a very large, beautifully decorated gazebo. Alexandra and Thomas had decided to do things a bit differently and had no bridesmaids or groomsmen. After the ceremony was over, everyone would walk over to the reception area which was nearby. They had tents set up that were open on the sides and had lovely decorated tables underneath. After pictures were done it wouldn't be long until sunset. Amy knew it was going to be gorgeous. It was a perfect day for an outdoor wedding and she was truly happy for her sister.

She suddenly felt a pang of sadness and tried to force it down. She and Jake had stood and said their vows and she remembered thinking what an amazing husband he was going to be. They had their struggles and tough times like any couple, but he had not let her down. The thing that made her sad was she had also thought on that day how she would be with this man for the rest of her life and he would be the father of her children and they would be grandparents together one day. Now that seemed like a dream somewhere far off. A sweet dream that she wished she could will herself to have each time she fell asleep but that seemed to elude her both in her dreams and her life.

She sighed and had no idea that tears had filled her eyes until Jake gently touched her arm. He leaned closer to her face and whispered, "Are you alright, Amy?" She then realized she could barely see him through her tears and worked at willing them away without letting any spill over and splash onto her cheeks. She forced a smile and nodded at him. He continued to study her eyes and she knew that he knew exactly what she was feeling. She could also see he wanted to hold her, but refrained. She knew it was not the time or place and was also grateful because if he even put his arm around her she knew the water works show to follow would not be stopped. She forced herself to think on other things and Jake wisely kept his distance and studied the wedding program.

After a few minutes had passed she turned to Jake and smiled. He looked relieved that she was herself again and flashed her a big smile of his own. Her heart thudded in an odd rhythm in her chest. His white teeth practically shown against his tanned skin and that combined with his dark hair and lovely dark eyes made him so strikingly handsome. She knew he would have this affect on her their entire lives. She felt like a teenager at the moment, but being the adult woman that she was wanted nothing more than to kiss the man she was married to. It was lovely that when she had those little surges of feelings that she could act on them rather than blush like a teenager who hadn't even yet revealed their crush for the other person. She settled for leaning over and kissing his cheek and whispering in his ear that he looked very good. His smile broadened and he said, "You're looking awfully good yourself, Mrs. Whitley."

She laughed lightly and then tucked her hand into the crook of his arm and looked at the wedding program with him.

Despite her hard work not long ago to focus on the event at hand and not on her own problems, her mind once again wandered to if she and Jake would ever have children. There were several here today including her little adorable niece, Suzie, who was sitting up a row and to Amy's left. As if she had read her Aunt's thoughts, Suzie turned around just then and flashed an endearing smile at Amy and waved. Amy's heart filled with love and longing all at once and it nearly took her breath away. Laura turned just then and flashed Jake and Amy a smile of her own and waved. Then she gently turned Suzie around to face the front.

Amy's emotion once again welled up and she felt her throat grow tight. *Oh Lord, will Jake and I ever sit at a wedding with our children?* She also had been noticing her sister's little, yet ever expanding, baby bump throughout the time they'd been here. *Will I ever have that Lord? Will I ever have our sweet baby growing inside of me? What does that feel like? Will I ever have a sweet little bundle who is Jake and I combined?* More thoughts and questions poured in her mind and she silently shared them all with her Heavenly Father.

She caught herself and realized she was going to be bawling in two seconds flat if she didn't make herself focus. She chided herself for allowing herself to grow emotional on this day. If she did cry, it needed to be tears of joy for her sister. She swallowed several times and was glad Jake was caught up in a conversation with the person seated on the other side of him. If he had looked at her just now, she would not have been able to hold herself together. She kept her feelings mostly to herself, but that man had her heart so completely that she could not only not hide anything from him, but he made her emotions come out more easily.

She fanned herself once again and made herself glance around again at the lovely decorations. She focused on the sounds of the birds chirping and the lovely hums of the gentle breeze and the soft music the two combined seemed to make. She felt relieved to once again have composure and told herself she would not allow thoughts of those kinds in her mind again tonight. This was Alex's day and she intended to focus on her and enjoy it.

Just then lovely piano music began and every one began talking in more hushed tones and began settling down for the ceremony. Jake turned to face the front and took her hand and gave it a gentle squeeze. He gave her a reassuring smile as if to say, "This is it. Your baby sister is getting married." So much joy filled her heart for Alexandra and it was hard to believe her little sister was about to be married. Didn't they talk and dream about their wedding days as little girls? Suddenly tears filled her eyes, but Amy did nothing to hide or fight them. She smiled as the tears gently streamed down her cheeks. Her little sister was getting married and it was a beautiful thing.

❤ ❤ ❤

Jadie had just gotten home from work and the scent of Oriental Lilies and Chrysanthemums was still quite prominent on her. So many people showered immediately when getting home from work due to being dirty or smelling like something that had to do with their vocation or sweat caused by it. Jadie smiled to herself that she came home smelling better than when she had left for work. Someone could literally say of her that she smelled like roses right after a day at work. She decided to change clothes later and got dinner preparations going. Once that was done and she had popped a pan of brownies in the oven for later, she decided to quickly check her e-mail while they baked.

These days it was very easy to "quickly" check her e-mail. When she had first joined her TTC Group, those e-mails had taken awhile to get through until she could figure out what was being said or she'd have to ask questions in response asking what something was as she wanted to learn. Now she could just quickly skim through them and catch exactly what was being said the first time. She was still learning about all the different medications and what they were used for, but other than that, for the most part she usually understood most of what was being said. It made her sad to think of how often someone would talk about something that was going on with them that she'd not heard of or women having to go through so many tests because their specialists couldn't figure out what was going on with them. So she was still learning things all the time, but as far as the abbreviation part of things and understanding much more about TTC in general, she was pretty well versed. The next e-mail she clicked on made her smile. When she had first joined it would have taken her forever to figure out what the woman was talking about and she wouldn't have even understood several of the things the woman referenced. But now, she read it with ease and understood everything.

"Well ladies, here is my update. I am on CD20. AF lasted a bit long this month, but we started doing the BD on CD9 just in case. I have been charting my BBT on FF as usual and that along with my OPK's are showing that I probably O'd around CD15. For those who don't remember, I don't O every month and was recently diagnosed with PCOS. But I have been taking Clomid to help with that, so I'm hoping to get my BFP soon. My CM and CP have been a little harder to chart this month as my body doesn't seem to be following it's usual pattern. Oh well, I'll just do my best! I am charting for me and also my RE wants me to so he can see how I'm responding to the meds. So now I'm in my 2ww and even though I'm only about 5 days in, I'm already dying to POAS! LOL. I am trying to hold off until I am at least 10DPO like a good girl. ;) I have just had so many BFN's and have a love/hate relationship with HPT's. I get so excited when I can finally test, but usually hate the result. Isn't that how it always goes? Anyways, send me and DH some baby dust! Good luck to the rest of you this month as well and congrats to those who have gotten their BFP's.

—Andrea"

Jadie typed out a quick response wishing her well this month and letting her know she was praying for her. Then she read the e-mail again aloud and was proud she could read it without once hesitating on any of the abbreviations.

"Well ladies, here is my update. I am on cycle day 20. Aunt Flow lasted a bit long this month, but we started doing the baby dance on cycle day 9 just in case. I have been charting my basal body temperature on Fertility Friend as usual and that along with my Ovulation Predictor Kits are showing that I probably ovulated around cycle day 15. For those who don't remember, I don't ovulate every month and was recently diagnosed with polycystic ovary syndrome. But I have been taking Clomid to help with that, so I'm hoping to get my big fat positive soon. My cervical mucus and cervical position have been a little harder to chart this month as my body doesn't seem to be following it's usual pattern. Oh well, I'll just do my best! I am charting for me and also my Reproductive Endocrinologist wants me to so he can see how I'm responding to the meds. So now I'm in my two week wait and even though I'm only about 5 days in, I'm already dying to pee on a stick! Laugh out loud. I am trying to hold off until I am at least ten days past ovulation like a good girl. I have just had so many big fat negatives and have a love/hate relationship with home pregnancy tests. I get so excited when I can finally test, but I usually hate the result. Isn't that how it always goes? Anyways, send me and dear husband some baby dust! Good luck to the rest of you this month as well as congrats to those who have gotten their big fat positives.

—Andrea"

Jadie totally related to what Andrea had shared about home pregnancy tests. She hated them as well because of the result they always gave her, but she too was often so eager to test that she could hardly stand it. When she had first joined the group, she had never heard of charting before. She had learned a lot about it since then though, and realized that a woman's basal body temperature could show where she was in her cycle and when she ovulated. She had found this fascinating! There was a really neat website that many of the girls on her group used called fertilityfriend.com that allowed them to keep track of that and all their other symptoms. Fertility Friend took all the data they entered and put it on a neat little chart that showed a graph of their temps along with abbreviations at the bottom to show their other symptoms and even medications they were taking on those days. Some women even checked their cervical position and entered it in their chart. Jadie found it all rather complicated and wasn't ready to do something like that yet, but she still found it very interesting!

The kitchen timer went off, so Jadie disconnected from the internet and headed to the kitchen. *Ahhh, the smell of brownies and flowers in the afternoon* she thought as she hummed. *It's good to be home, sweet home.*

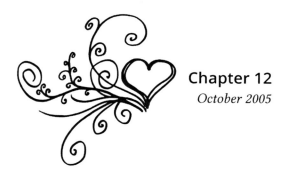

Chapter 12
October 2005

J adie wanted to feel optimistic, but the one year
mark was quickly approaching and she feared they
would reach it. She reflected back on how badly she
had felt for all the women on her group who were dealing with
infertility months back and how she couldn't imagine how that
felt. Suddenly she did know how it felt and she had a feeling in
her heart that she would soon be counted among them. In a way
she felt stunned. She just hardly ever heard of anyone having
trouble with it and it had always seemed kind of rare. When they
had started trying it never entered her mind that it may take a
long time or even not work out for them. That just always seemed
like something you didn't hear about often and that happened
to someone else. But now she was the someone else. She also
wrongly assumed that infertility ran in families and had learned
that was most often not the case. She daily had to squelch feelings
that tried to rise up and cloud her mind with an intense fog of
negative thoughts like "it's never going happen," "you will never
have children," "you're broken," "your heart's deepest desire will
never be fulfilled," "you will never watch your family grow or
be a grandmother," and on and on it went. Some days it felt like
she was in an actual battle to keep those things out of her mind.

Suddenly it seemed as though her eyes focused on what

they were actually seeing starting from her peripheral vision and moving towards the center. The beautiful colors of the trees whizzing by came into view. She couldn't help but sigh as she saw God's handiwork before her. She loved this time of year. The air seemed crisper and cleaner somehow and that combined with the beautiful colors always made her admire the season and what God had created. Chase was quiet in the seat next to her. They were driving to a larger town about a half an hour away to pick up some tools and supplies Chase needed for work and to get some groceries and maybe even do some early Christmas shopping.

Had it really been a year? Time had seemed to drag on forever while they waited and on the other hand still seemed to somehow speed by. It had felt like they'd been waiting a long time, but at the same time, it felt crazy that it was almost a year since it had all begun.

She voiced her feelings to her husband and he merely nodded with a sad look on his face.

"What are you thinking, Chase?"

He sighed. "Just how badly I want to be a daddy and how bad I want to make your dream come true."

"You say that like you're hindering it somehow."

"Sometimes I feel like I am. Like something is wrong with me. Like maybe I don't work right and what if I can't give you what you want? I know you'll still love me, but it'll always feel like it's my fault."

Jadie reached over and took his hand. She was nearly broken hearted by his admission. "Oh, honey. There is nothing wrong with you and even if something were physically wrong, it would never be your fault."

Chase glanced at her and then back at the road. She had said it with such conviction and also laced with pain that he knew she meant it.

"I know. I can't help but feel like that sometimes though."

"I know what you mean. Ultimately though, God is in control and it's no one's fault. 'So are My ways higher than your ways

And My thoughts than your thoughts'." She ended by quoting part of the verses from Isaiah 55:8 and 9 that they always reminded each other of to encourage each other.

He smiled slightly and squeezed her hand. "Yeah, it's in His hands."

Jadie bristled and forced the thought from her mind. The one that often came out of the blue and plagued her. If it was in God's hands, why did He allow them to suffer? She made herself remember that it was humans' fault, ever since the fall that happened in the garden of Eden, that things with the world were not always right. God had created everything and everyone perfect. It was sin that caused things, including people's bodies, to not always work the way they should. And that we all live in a fallen world broken by sin. Still, she knew He had the power to fix what was going on with them and give them a baby and He didn't. She reminded herself again of the verse she had just quoted to Chase. God knew what He was doing and she was just going to have to trust Him whether she wanted to or not.

A song came on the radio just then that reminded Jadie of a song someone from her TTC group had told her about. It was called "I Would Die for That" by Kellie Coffey. Jadie had looked up the music video on YouTube and proceeded to bawl her eyes out. She felt like it could be her theme song. When Chase had gotten home, she'd had him watch as well. He too was deeply moved by it and just held her as they watched. Their broken hearts seemed united with that of the singer and all the people who had gone through or were still going through infertility as they watched. Like they all had one thing in common that they completely understood each other on, regardless of anything else in their personalities or lives. It connected them to each other in a very real way. Jadie could still hear all the powerful words combined with the moving music in her head and reflected on them again.

"Jenny was my best friend.
Went away one summer.
Came back with a secret
She just couldn't keep.
A child inside her,
Was just too much for her
So she cried herself to sleep.
And she made a decision
Some find hard to accept.
Too young to know that one day
She might live to regret.

But I would die for that.
Just to have one chance
To hold in my hands
All that she had.
I would die for that.

I've been given so much,
A husband that I love.
So why do I feel incomplete?
With every test and checkup
We're told not to give up.
He wonders if it's him.
And I wonder if it's me.

All I want is a family,
Like everyone else I see.
And I won't understand it
If it's not meant to be.

Cause I would die for that.
Just to have one chance
To hold in my hands
All that they have.
I would die for that.

And I want to know what it's like
To bring a dream to life.
For that kind of love,
What I'd give up!
I would die for that.

Sometimes it's hard to conceive,
With all that I've got,
And all I've achieved,
What I want most
Before my time is gone,
Is to hear the words "I love you, Mom."

I would die for that.
Just to have one chance
To hold in my hands
What so many have.
I would die for that.
And I want to know what it's like
To bring a dream to life.
How I would love
What some give up. I would die . . .
I would die for that."

♥ ♥ ♥

The pile of books that needed to be put back on the shelves, in alphabetical order of course, seemed especially monstrous today. The library seemed particularly busy today and Amy found herself checking the clock frequently. Two more hours and she could go home! She could hardly wait. There had been an abnormal amount of people checking out books today and that left Amy behind on some of her other duties, so she was rushing to catch up in between helping people check out books. There was finally a lull and she had sorted most of the returned books into stacks according to section. She grabbed an armful of two sections and headed off to try to get as many placed back in their spots as she could before someone else needed her help.

The distraction was good for her she was sure. She had been having more hot flashes from being on the Clomid lately and it was difficult to not let their situation consume her thoughts. So far the Clomid hadn't worked, at least enough to result in a pregnancy, but she reassured herself that they still had time.

Jake had been busy lately too. Although he had been for awhile now. She was glad that her husband did such a great job of still making so much time for her despite often working overtime and with his classes and studying towards becoming an electrician. He would continue to work where he did presently, but it would give him a substantial promotion within the company along with more benefits and a hefty raise. Amy couldn't be prouder of him. If all went well, he should be taking his final exams not even a year from now. In a way, it still felt like a long ways off.

As Amy slid book after book back onto the shelves and felt accomplishment to see the pile shrinking, she thought, as she often did, of all the girls from her TTC group. She tried to remember as many names as she could and she silently prayed for them as she worked. Some of them were having harder times than others, some were going through difficult treatments, some had decided to just try naturally and hoped and waited month after month, new people joined, some finally got their "BFP's" and most of them left the group shortly after, and on and on it went. Amy's heart both rejoiced and sank when she saw those three letters show up in the subject line of her e-mails sometimes. She was elated that someone had finally gotten their amazing news, but her heart could not help but cry out, "Will it ever be my turn?"

Amy thought about how her sister Laura had been a great listening ear and compassionate heart to Amy since she'd shared the news of their infertility and PCOS diagnosis a few months ago. Laura didn't know what to say oftentimes, but Amy had told her what things bothered her when they were said and Laura was amazing about never bringing that up again. Even though her sister hadn't been through it personally, she was very supportive, sensitive, and Amy knew Laura prayed for her often. When Laura had shared that she was pregnant and had held off on telling for awhile due to Amy's news, it had touched Amy deeply. She was genuinely happy for her sister, but she had days where it was a hard and painful reminder of what she lacked as well. All in all Amy felt happy she'd told because it gave her someone to talk to in person who had known her for her whole life and it also had strengthened their already close bond which was a blessing in many ways.

The pile continued to shrink and Amy chuckled to herself that this was a time in her day that her work wasn't really distracting her at all, but gave her time to think about it all. She supposed that wasn't necessarily a bad thing. She did wish she could think about it less, but that just didn't seem possible.

Amy realized that she and Jadie now talked some way or another to each other a good four times a week at least. They talked on the phone fairly often and also e-mailed frequently and had "instant messaging dates." Amy was still amazed at how quickly they had formed a bond and how close they were, especially considering that Amy was usually a very private person. But she supposed that God had brought them to each other because He knew they needed one another. She was very glad He had! She marveled at how He often gave His children just what they needed. She thought, not for the first time, about how God didn't promise His children wouldn't have hardships, just that He'd be there with them along the way. It was a beautiful reminder to Amy that God loved her and kept all His promises.

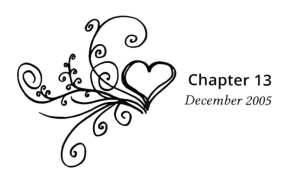

Chapter 13
December 2005

Christmas decorations were everywhere. Ones for inside and outside, some small and some large, some inexpensive and some very expensive. Jadie held tighter to Chase's hand with her left and stuffed her right hand deep into the pocket of her favorite pea coat. Jadie loved everything about Christmas and had never been in a store like this before. Chase had decided to take her out on a date night and this was one of the stops. It did lighten Jadie's mood and make her happy, but reminders of what they were missing seemed to scream at her from nearly every shelf. She let her eyes linger on a tiny stocking that said "Baby's First Christmas." She drug her eyes away and looked at other things, determined to be happy tonight.

Chase squeezed her hand and gave her a knowing look. He had seen the stocking too.

Jadie gave him a sad smile in return and squeezed his hand back. No words were needed. Her husband understood her heart and felt the pain too and that was enough comfort for now.

Chase let go of her hand and rushed over to a wreath made completely of Christmas tree bulbs. He reminded her of a little boy as he said excitedly, "Look at this, Jadie! This would be perfect for above the fireplace. What do you think?"

She walked over and admired it up close. "I do really like it!"

She looked at all the beautiful colors of bulbs and saw her reflection in one of them. Her face looked slightly distorted and her image reflected back was tinged by the color of the bulb. Jadie's shoulders slumped a little. She found it very fitting. She felt like infertility distorted and tinged everything she saw, felt, and experienced these days. She sighed without realizing it.

Chase looked at her, concern etching his expression. "What's wrong honey? Don't you like it?"

Jadie tucked both hands in her pockets and blew out a breath. "No, it's not that. I love it. It'd be great above the fireplace … like you said."

Chase leaned a bit to get her attention so she would turn her eyes towards him. Once she did he replied, "Well, then what's wrong?"

She sighed again. "What is always wrong. I feel so frustrated at myself. It feels like it's all I can think about some days." She went on to explain what she felt when she saw her reflection in the bulb.

Chase's expression was sad as he said, "I understand. Take comfort in knowing you're not alone. I really do understand honey. I have a really hard time with it too. I don't always experience the exact same thoughts or feelings, but not having a baby on the way yet feels like it's killing me at times. I hoped tonight would get our minds off of it. But I suppose that was silly. Not having what we so desperately want makes that stand out all the more in places like this. A huge part of Christmas is family and tradition." His voice grew even more sad and quiet. "And it feels like we have a hole in our family right now."

Jadie's lip quivered and her eyes brimmed with tears. She looked at him and nodded and then looked away so she could compose herself. That man saw straight through to her soul when she looked at him and she would really lose it if she kept looking into his kind and loving eyes. Finally she took a deep breath and answered him. "It's good to know you understand. It is really hard, but I'm at least glad we're in it together." She reached out and took his hand. He offered her a weak smile and then looked back down towards his shoes.

She doubled her resolve and playfully swung her arm back and forth. She forced her voice to be upbeat as she said, "Alright now, Mr. Taylor, we have a lot of store yet to get through before dinner. This was a great idea and I am really glad we came. Let's look and have fun."

She watched as the sparkle mostly returned to her husband's eyes. "Alright, Mrs. Taylor, let's get shopping!"

On the car ride on the way home, Jadie watched the different groupings of stores pass by and the way the snow fell softly and was illuminated brighter in certain spots by the street lamps. She thought about what a pretty scene it made. But still her heart felt weighted down. Last month marked a year since they had started trying for her and Chase. They had talked about it a lot and it had been a rough time for both of them. Jadie felt like she now had no choice but to accept reality. She had heard on her TTC group plenty of times and saw tons of times during her online research what one year of unprotected sex meant. An automatic infertility diagnosis. She had tried so hard to fight fear and doubt as it had crowded around her and threatened to suffocate her so many times over the past thirteen months. But she couldn't hide any longer. Something she thought she would never face or experience was here and she had to face it. She and Chase were going through infertility.

They had prayed a lot about it and had briefly mentioned going to an infertility specialist a couple of times. Jadie had never been able to imagine what she would do were she to be in this situation . . . until now. She and Chase both agreed that they would take whatever steps necessary to have a biological child. They thought adoption was a wonderful thing and that was definitely on their radar as well. But they both knew they wanted a child of their own . . . no matter what. They would go all the way to surrogacy if they needed to. Jadie remembered telling Chase over a year ago how amazing it was that a baby of their's would be him and her combined into one tiny little person. How much closer could two people get than God actually putting them together to make another person who was half of each of them? They had been a little quiet so far on the ride home and she decided to talk to Chase about it.

"I had a lot of fun tonight, honey. Thank you."

He glanced briefly in her direction. "You're welcome. I had a really nice time too."

Jadie loved the way the snow looked like millions of shooting stars coming gently towards the windshield. She allowed a moment to pass and then said, "I don't want to ruin our evening, but . . ."

Once again Chase cautiously glanced at her for the briefest of moments and then flipped the right turn signal on and gently turned right at a light. "But what?"

"Do you mind if we talk about . . . you know." she asked tentatively.

"No honey, I don't mind. It's a big part of our life right now. We have to talk about it when either of us wants or needs to. That doesn't mean it'll ruin tonight. Go ahead."

She loved how wonderful and understanding he was and felt confident to forge ahead. "Well, we just haven't talked much about seeing an infertility specialist and I was wondering what your thoughts were about that."

"You mean going now?"

"Well, just your thoughts in general. I know we both want to go at some point and since we have hit the one year mark now, I was just wondering if you felt we should go soon or if we should wait."

Chase nodded thoughtfully and kept his eyes on the road. He was driving rather slowly and being cautious because of the snow so it would take them longer to get home, but Jadie didn't mind. It was a beautiful night and gave them more time to talk. She also enjoyed spending even the most ordinary moments like this with her husband. She cherished the small things in life.

"I really would like to go and find out what's going on, but I'm just nervous about our finances. Winter is a slower time for my job and I just don't know how much that all is going to cost. We are a little behind right now, so I am just not sure if it's the best timing."

Jadie had thought about this same thing, but her heart still sunk to hear her husband say it aloud. In most states, infertility was not covered by insurance and their's was no exception.

"I know. I've thought about that too. It's so hard to know what to do! When do you dive in and just trust God to take care of things and when do you use the brain He gave you and try to be wise about when to do certain things?"

Chase well understood the frustration in his wife's voice at that last part. "That was a perfect way to put it! I often wonder where the line between faith in diving in and using discernment in decision making is."

They both sighed at the same time and then found themselves laughing.

Jadie said, "It's a pickle, that's for sure."

Chase raised his eyebrows high on his head and let them drop again and gave a shake of his head. "It sure is! I think the best we can do for now is to just really pray about it. We will together at night when we usually pray, but we'll both pray individually too. Hopefully we'll feel God leading us one way or another. And in the meantime we'll try to pinch our pennies the best we can and catch up and then maybe even start saving a little."

Jadie knew that could take some time, but the confidence in her husband's sound plan did her heart good. She put her gloved hand in his as they were presently on a road that had been snow plowed bare, and told him that she loved both ideas and that's just what they'd do.

♥ ♥ ♥

Jadie rushed back into the sanctuary of her church to grab her Bible case. She had been visiting and set it down to hug someone and then forgotten all about it. "Good, still here." she said quietly to herself as she picked it up. She was glad no one had taken it to the lost and found yet.

She turned and had only taken a few steps when an older woman who she had known for years walked up.

"Hi Jadie. How are you?"

Jadie flashed her a warm smile. "Good Mrs. Anderson. How are you?"

"I am well, thanks. Hank has a cold today and stayed home."

"Oh, well I'm sorry to hear that. I guess it's been going around."

"It has at that! So how is Chase's work going?"

"Oh, pretty well. This is kind of their slow season, but they're hanging in there."

"Well, hopefully after the new year things will pick up again."

"Yes, I hope so!"

Right then a couple of children ran by who were about five or six years old. Both women watched them rush past and smiled and shook their heads.

Mrs. Anderson said, "Oh to have half their energy."

Jadie laughed. "Isn't that the truth?"

"So when are you and Chase going to have some little bundles of energy?" she said warmly and with a smile.

Jadie felt the blood drain from her face and felt the familiar cold feeling that spread through her whenever someone asked her that.

She gave the practiced and perfunctory answer that she always did when asked questions like this and prayed her voice sounded normal. "Well, Chase and I got married fairly young and we just wanted to enjoy some time to ourselves, get settled in a home, and save up some before having children. We always said we'd wait a few years." She forced a smile that she didn't feel and could tell her lips were wobbly. It was the truth, she was always just vague on the timeframe and neglected to share that they felt they'd waited long enough.

"I see. Well that's very sensible of you, dear. I think it's wise to enjoy some time just being married before having children. Waiting a good five years at least would be really great."

Jadie fought down the frustration building in her. This was how it always was. Someone asked the question with such expectation and with an obvious hint of "what's the hold up?" to their voice or in their expression (or both) and then when she answered, they always ended up saying that she and Chase were right and should wait even longer or some other opinion. Some people expressed it stronger than others, but Jadie just felt people were too opinionated one way or the other. She knew that Mrs. Anderson was just trying to make conversation, but it was just tough. It felt like no one approved of the time frame either way! Not to mention every time someone asked them why they didn't have a baby yet or when they were going to be trying, Jadie felt like someone was stabbing her heart with a knife. Didn't people know how hard this was without the probing questions, painful reminders, and then unwanted advice and opinions given? Jadie scolded herself. Of course they didn't know, because no one had any idea what they were going through anyways. But even though people didn't know, it didn't change the fact that it still was frustrating and it still hurt . . . badly. Jadie also had heard enough on her TTC group to know that even if you did tell people, no one seemed to understand. Poor Amy was another prime example of that in Jadie's mind.

Jadie shook her head. Even though only a few heartbeats had passed, it felt like longer. "Well, Mrs. Anderson, it was so nice to see you, but I best be finding Chase and getting home."

"Oh yes dear. Nice to see you as well. I best get home to Hank anyways."

"Tell him we said hi and that we want him to get well."

"Thank you. I will!"

Jadie gave her a nod and resisted the urge to run from the sanctuary and made herself walk as normally as possible. She couldn't wait to get home.

Later that afternoon, Jadie was thrilled when the phone rang and she heard Amy's voice on the other line when she answered. She had said she may call and Jadie was so glad she had! After small talk, they discussed what had happened at church. Amy was very understanding as always and Jadie felt calmer after having talked with her about it. Jadie sometimes worried she was being overly sensitive at times, but after reading her e-mails or talking to Amy, she realized that what they were going through was just very tough and painful and it was difficult to not have strong feelings about it. Jadie was so glad she could vent to Amy and her group and they always understood so well. Of course she talked to Chase about everything too, but it was always nice to have other women from all walks of life who also understood her pain. Suddenly Jadie remembered something she had wanted to ask Amy. Chase was napping on the couch and she knew he would be okay with her talking to Amy about it, but it made it easier for Jadie since he couldn't hear her talking to her friend about something so personal.

"Ummm . . . Amy?"

"Yeah?"

"Can I ask you something . . . well, personal?"

Amy chuckled. "Of course! You should know by now that in the world of TTC nothing is off limits! Especially with me."

Jadie smiled, but she still felt nervous asking. "Well, is it sometimes hard to . . . how do you deal with . . . well, what I mean to say is . . . "

Amy replied in a soothing and more serious tone, "Go ahead . . . you can ask me."

"Well, is it sometimes hard to keep the intimacy in your marriage feeling . . . natural and sporadic when sometimes it has to be so planned and it feels kind of forced?"

"Oh absolutely! It can be a real challenge to keep things feeling normal when you feel like 'this is the day, whether we feel like it or not!' " She laughed. "It takes a real effort to try to keep things from becoming all business and losing the romantic and special part of it."

Jadie audibly sighed. "I'm so glad it's not just me! You worded it so well! Sometimes it does seem like it's just all business and it can be hard. I don't want that part of our marriage to suffer because of our infertility."

"I know just what you mean. Just keep working at it and do your best to not let the schedule take over everything."

"It's just such a challenge sometimes. I mean, we're willing to try anything to help and it's just not super romantic to say, 'Hey, hold on a second while I put a pillow under my butt.'" Amy laughed outright and very hard. Her friend's frustrated and matter-of-fact tone on top of what she said made Amy not be able to hold back. She wasn't laughing at Jadie and she was relieved when her friend joined her in laughing so she knew she hadn't hurt her feelings.

"I know just what you mean!"

"I'm sorry if that was graphic, but I actually feel relieved that you laughed! It's nice to know someone gets it and can even find the crazy things that we do to try to help things along humorous."

"You weren't being graphic. I have seen the girls suggest that many, many times on the group. That along with certain positions and all kinds of other things to help. Infertility can definitely get personal, but hey, that's the way you make a baby! And sometimes you need to be able to laugh at certain aspects of it."

"Yeah, it does feel nice to have someone who completely understands and can laugh with you."

"Yes, it really is."

Jadie went on to tell Amy that she had ordered FertiliAid off the internet for her and Chase to try. It was an all-natural vitamin that she'd heard about on the group that could help regulate some things in the body naturally to help aid fertility.

"Oh, that's good! Jake and I use that as well. It's not very expensive and it can't hurt."

"That's what Chase and I figured."

Amy added, "Since we've been on the topic of personal, there is also a lubricant I wonder if you've heard about. They talk about it on the group sometimes. There are no harmful chemicals in it to harm the sperm and in fact it is supposed to help their motility and increase your chances in several ways."

"I have heard about it on the group. Do you have the website?"

They talked about that for a few more minutes and then moved onto other topics before hanging up a short time later. Jadie touched her cheeks with her palms and realized she still had a slight blush and warmth to her cheeks from the direction of some of their conversation. At the same time, she smiled. It felt so wonderful to have someone to talk to about all of this. Like Amy said, the very nature of trying to make a baby was quite personal. Sometimes it needed to be talked about if you needed advice or something to aid your efforts and that was okay.

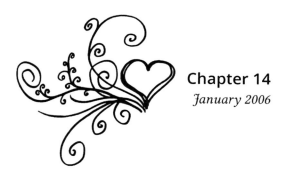

Chapter 14
January 2006

The negative sign on the pregnancy test practically screamed at Amy. It felt very final and sad. Six months had went by since Amy had been on Clomid and the dreaded two week wait was over. She'd taken the test and the symbol she had seen so many times before and could seem to find no escape from, had shown up for her yet again. She sighed as she sat on the edge of the tub. She threw the test in the trash can and looked over at Jake who had been pacing by the sink. His fist was over his mouth and under his nose and the look on his face said everything that Amy was feeling and she was sure she looked the same way. She didn't have to say anything, he knew from her reaction the news wasn't good. He took her hand and pulled her up and hugged her. She found comfort even in feeling his warm breath on her hair.

She pulled away slightly and looked up at him. She asked him the question that she didn't want to wait to ask; she wanted to keep moving. "What now?"

He released her and took her hand and led her to the couch where they both flopped down rather dejectedly.

She waited for his deep voice to resonate in their small living room as he spoke. He cleared his throat and then said, "Well, we've talked about this some in the past. How far we were willing to go I mean. Before we even knew about your PCOS, we said we'd be willing to go pretty far. Do you still feel that way?"

She knew the answer in her heart and didn't even hesitate, but nodded fervently.

He tipped his head back against the couch and looked at the ceiling. "So do I." He paused and then said, "Well, Dr. Moyer said the next step she would recommend would be IUI. We've discussed this and money isn't something that's going to stop us. But do you feel up to that Amy? That's going to be a lot on you physically and a lot of pressure for us both emotionally. Is that what we want to do?"

The way they did so often it seemed ever since their journey through infertility had started, Amy's eyes filled with tears. She hated it, but did nothing to hide the emotion from her husband. "I know it will be hard, but we both agree we want to do more. So if that's the next step, then I say let's go for it. Let's exhaust all our options. I am not at peace to stop until we try everything we feel we should."

Jake listened intently and then solemnly nodded. "I agree. We had said we would do IUI even a couple of times if it came to that. How many times do you think we should try?"

She quickly said, "I don't want to do anything you're not comfortable with."

He shook his head. "Have you been praying about it?"

"I have."

"So have I. Let's just say the number we both feel like would be right for us. If it's the same number, great. If not, then we can discuss it and try to come up with what we both feel is best. Okay?"

Amy bit her lip and nodded.

"Okay, on three. One ... two ... three ..."

"Two." "Two." was said simultaneously.

Amy's eyes grew a little wide. Jake couldn't help but think she looked adorable and smiled a little. "Well, I guess that decision is made. We're on the same page."

Amy smiled a little too. "Okay, well I'll call Dr. Moyer tomorrow and make an appointment and we can go from there."

"Alright."

"Should we maybe . . . what would you think about . . ."

"What is it, Amy?"

"Well, I know it's a lot to take in all in one day and we're making a lot of decisions, but I find peace in having a plan and knowing where we're going. There were just so many months of uncertainty and I like that we just keep diving right in."

"I agree completely. So what else are you thinking of? I think I might know, but go ahead and tell me."

"Well, we had talked about adoption too and I know from when we researched it some awhile back that it can take some time. I was just wondering if we should make a decision on that as well."

Jake thought for a moment. "You mean on how to pursue it?"

"Yes. From talking last time, I know we were leaning towards foster care. I am just wondering if we should decide how we want to pursue that option and then maybe get the ball rolling since it can take some time. But I know you have a lot going on right now as it is with work and studying . . ." Jake held up his hand to stop her.

"There is nothing more important to me than growing our family." He turned towards her and took both of her smaller hands into his own. Amy loved how strong they were and how his hand covered her entire hand. Even though they were so strong, he couldn't have been more gentle. He made her feel so loved and safe. She focused on his earnest face and listened. "I don't feel like I will be stressed out too much if we start another process. That was already popping into my mind at the same time I think it was your's. We had talked about that in the past and also that it's something we would consider pursuing even if we have a baby of our own. So I think it may be wise to get that process going as well and even if we do conceive on our own, we will already have that going even if we wouldn't take any children for awhile."

Amy nodded. "So I guess we need to decide for sure if we

want to do foster care and look into agencies in the area then."

Jake's deep voice felt like it covered her with a thick velvet of comfort and assurance.

"I think we should pray together and then how about Friday night we start doing some homework and maybe even make some calls."

Amy nodded. "That sounds good."

Jake smiled. "Good. It's a date then."

He leaned forward and hugged her again and they prayed together for the first time about the specific situation they now found themselves in.

They continued to pray separately and together and on Friday night they had their "homework date." By the end of the evening they had made two big decisions. They were pursuing foster care and they had already found their agency. They knew God was answering their prayers. Now it was just a matter of waiting to see what resulted from both pursuits: IUI and foster care.

♥ ♥ ♥

Pine needles lay scattered all over the living room floor and Jadie went to get her vacuum cleaner to sweep them up. She loved the holidays. Tradition, good food, time with family, and everything else surrounding that time of year always made her very happy. But these days it also made her wonder if or when she and Chase would get to start more traditions with their own little family or have a little one to take to gatherings. Finn and Sarah's little boy, Charlie, was getting so big. Jadie loved her nephew immensely, but he also made her feel a hole in her heart that nothing seemed to fill. It wasn't his fault of course and she didn't not want to spend time with him because of it, but it was hard sometimes. Sarah was also expecting another baby. Jadie reflected back on how at both Christmas and New Years celebrations on Chase's side she had asked Sarah if she could touch her belly. Jadie felt in awe and wonder as her little niece rolled around and kicked in there. She could watch and feel Sarah's stomach all day long. It was the neatest thing! Sarah also had new ultrasound pictures to share. Tears had filled Jadie's eyes when she saw such sweet and perfect little feet and toes and hands and fingers. She also loved the classic profile shot where she could see her perfect little face and adorable rounded tummy. Jadie ached so badly to know what it would feel like to be pregnant and to go to her own ultrasounds. It seemed like it would the most wonderful thing in the world to think about, but to her it was tainted by pain as she wondered if it would ever happen for her and since it felt like a wonderful dream that was just out of her grasp.

Jadie wiped her nose and sniffed and realized she was kneeling by the needles on her floor crying and not moving. She quickly plugged in the vacuum and swept up the last visible traces of their Christmas tree. She always hated taking it down each year. Earlier this morning she had taken all the other Christmas decorations from their home and packed them neatly into their boxes and put them in the closet until next year. Once she had put the vacuum away, she felt satisfaction at a project done and seeing her house all tidy. She headed to the bathroom to freshen up before heading over to her mom's house. She had decided to go over there today and spend some time with her mom and then Chase would come straight there from work so they could all have dinner together once her dad got home as well.

When Jadie got to her mom's, she greeted her with a warm hug and then they visited while sharing some hot chocolate and eating some snacks still left over from the holidays. Jadie had fun just talking with her mom and after they cleaned up a bit in the kitchen they headed to the living room to visit. Jadie had rented a chick flick for them to watch before the guys got home and looked forward to watching it. They were talking about the holidays when her mom said, "I just can't wait until we have grandbabies in the family as well to celebrate with. It'll just be so fun!" Her mom had a big smile and a wistful look on her face until she turned to Jadie and saw her daughter's serious expression.

"What is it, honey?" her mom asked with concern.

Jadie was so tired of hiding this from her mom. They were really close and shared most everything with each other. She and Chase had originally decided to keep their TTC to themselves because it felt personal and they didn't want people asking them how it was going all the time. They also thought it would be fun to surprise every one with the news once it happened since no one would be expecting it. Knowing what she did now, Jadie was infinitely grateful that they'd kept things to themselves. At the same time, Jadie had begun to long to share it with someone. Having her TTC group and Amy to talk to was wonderful of course, but she wanted to share it with those close to her too. Chase had said she could tell whomever whenever she wanted as long as they kept it in confidence since he knew it was important for Jadie to be able to talk to people about it. He preferred to keep it to himself, however, and they both respected the way each other felt about it.

Her mom reached out and gently touched her arm. "Honey?"

Jadie licked her lips. Should she just go ahead and tell her? She'd been contemplating it for a little while now. She felt safe to do so and made a quick decision to tell her mom.

She looked up and then shyly looked back down at her hands that she'd just folded in her lap. "It would be great to have some little ones in the family." She paused for a moment. "Speaking of that, there's something I want to tell you."

Her mom's face had become drawn with concern. "What is it, dear?"

Jadie felt her palms grow sweaty although she felt cold. Even though she felt close to her mother, it still didn't feel easy to share. "Well . . . Chase and I have been trying to have a baby for about fourteen months now, but so far, it hasn't been working."

There. She'd said it. She felt relief in a way, but was also anxious to see what her mom would have to say about it. She glanced up at her mom and forced her eyes to stay there.

Her mom's shock was evident on her face. "Oh honey. Why didn't you tell me?"

The compassion in her voice made Jadie's throat grow thick from the sudden onset of tears.

"Well, it just felt personal and we ..." she let her voice trail off.

Her mom nodded. "Yes, I suppose your dad and I didn't announce when we were trying to have a baby. I just wish I had known. It's obviously painful for you and I wish I could have helped somehow."

Jadie's tears were very close now and she just pressed her lips tight together and shook her head.

Her mom reached for her and held her while Jadie let some tears roll down her cheeks. Being hugged by her momma did her heart a world of good.

Finally she pulled back and took a deep breath. "I would appreciate it if you could be praying for us."

"Of course, honey! Daddy and I both will be." She wouldn't admit it to Jadie, but she just felt stunned by this news. She had never had trouble conceiving, so why was Jadie? She decided to voice a question she did have though.

"Have you and Chase considered seeing a doctor?"

Jadie nodded. "We have, but we're just praying and saving our money for now."

Keira nodded thoughtfully. "I see."

Jadie watched her mother a moment and then said, "Are you thinking anything mom? You seem quiet."

Keira gave Jadie's hand a few gentle pats and offered a small, reassuring smile. "Oh, I am just a little surprised and am just thinking is all."

Jadie nodded again.

Keira had so many questions racing through her head, so she asked Jadie a few. Jadie answered them easily and then Keira thought again for a moment.

"You know, I can see you're really upset about this and I don't blame you. Any parent hates to see their child suffering, but ..."

Jadie didn't know why, but she stiffened and braced herself. "But what?"

"But I just wonder if you're thinking about this too much. Stress can really have a strong impact on our bodies and maybe you and Chase are just stressing over it too much. Maybe just relax, you know . . . let it happen. I've even heard of people who went away on vacation for awhile and then got pregnant. It seems to help when people relax."

Jadie's entire body was now rigid and she clenched her fists so tight that her nails dug into her palms. She knew her mom was trying to help, but did she seriously just tell her to "let it happen"? As if Jadie was stopping it from happening? She had heard all the stories too of people getting pregnant while on vacation, but she couldn't help but feel a strong frustration. Were people really so naive as to think that a vacation actually helped someone get pregnant when they were having problems?

Jadie took a deep breath. "I realize, mom, that stress isn't good for a person. But I didn't go into this stressed. I started stressing after it wasn't working. And Chase and I aren't trying to be uptight or stressed about it. It's just a little hard when we don't know if we'll ever have children." She made herself look down for a moment to compose herself.

"I didn't think about it like that–that you didn't go into it stressed. I guess I've just heard people say that a lot over the years."

Jadie sighed. "I know. That seems to be a common belief."

Keira couldn't help but notice the annoyance laced in her daughter's voice. "And honey, you'll have children. You'll see."

The pain on Jadie's face as she looked up at her nearly took her breath away. "How do you know, momma? I might not."

Keira suddenly felt very choked up. "I think it will happen, honey. Just hang in there."

They sat quietly for a moment and then Keira asked, "Why did you say that was a common belief? The stress thing, I mean."

Jadie rolled her eyes. "Because everyone says that. I am on a group online for women who are trying to conceive. Every single person on there has been told that by people they share it with. And unless they're brave enough to share their feelings on that and ask people not to say that to them, people just keep on saying it. So please don't say that to me mom. I am not making myself not get pregnant because I'm stressed. Infertility is caused by something not being right physically with our bodies. It's not a psychologically caused hindrance."

Keira took a moment to let that sink in. She had never thought about it much, but in every situation she could reflect back on now, it did seem that every one she knew had always said that about people who struggled to get pregnant. But she'd also never thought of it from Jadie's perspective either. Her daughter had good points.

She licked her lips. "I see what you're saying and it is strange that so many of us seem to think that same thing. But maybe there is some merit to it. I was just watching a show the other day and they were showing all the negative effects stress can have on people and . . ."

Jadie couldn't take it any longer. She already felt very emotional for some reason today and now she'd shared this with her mother and was already being berated by the stupid stress comments! She wanted compassion, not theories that made it seem as though Jadie herself caused this to happen!

She raised her voice even though she didn't want to. "Mom! Just stop, ok? I realize stress isn't good; I'm not a complete idiot! But I did not cause this to happen because it eventually effected my emotions! Chase and I are not trying to be stressed. But that's like telling someone who has cancer to not have any feelings about it. 'Don't be stressed!' 'Don't think about it too much.' 'If you weren't so stressed out, maybe you'd get better.' No! Someone who has cancer did not cause it by being stressed that they may get cancer. It just happened and then they get stressed. It's the same with infertility! I wasn't worrying about it not happening. It never even entered my mind that we might not be able to get pregnant easily until we didn't get pregnant for months on end!

Then the stress began. So you see how that's in the wrong order for it to have caused it?"

Keira's mouth gaped open. Her daughter hadn't raised her voice to her since she was a teenager. She quickly tried to think of what to say to calm down her very upset daughter. She said in a very kind voice, "Honey, I'm sorry if I implied you caused this. I didn't mean it like that, I just meant that maybe it's hindering things now is all. Maybe you should go on vacation just to get away from all this for awhile. Or have you thought about adopting? You know my aunt's cousin and her husband did that after trying for like ten years and then got pregnant. Or . . ."

Jadie jumped off the couch and raised her voice even more. Her eyes were large and she had a very frustrated look on her face. She felt so infuriated inside for all the thousands of times that people going through infertility had heard this. It didn't help that recently on her group there had been even more stories than normal about people getting insensitive comments. It was probably due to the holidays. Even people who had shared their struggles were still asked "When are you guys going to have kids?" Some were even told ridiculous and cruel things like they didn't want it enough. One woman had shared that her sister-in-law had told her, "Why don't you take my kids for a day, that'll cure you from wanting your own" and someone else was told to "be grateful" that they didn't have the added expense of having a child around the holidays. All this was on Jadie's mind and then to have her mom parrot the same ridiculous theories that everyone with infertility seemed to hear over and over . . . it was just too much and she snapped.

"Seriously mom? You think if we adopt then we'll magically get pregnant? Why does every one share these stories? Did everyone on the earth take a class of ridiculous theories to share with people who are having trouble having kids? Why does every one think that stress causes it and adoption will fix it? Did anyone ever consider that after trying to get pregnant the next step for that couple was to adopt a baby? And that then God just gave them a miracle? Do people seriously believe that adoption can cause someone to get pregnant? What kind of logic is that? That makes absolutely no sense to me! God makes babies, okay, God does. And He does it when He wants. So are there stories of people getting pregnant after adopting a child? Uh, yeah, duh! A lot of people adopt while they are still trying and then something works out or God just gives them a miracle. Just because someone had a biological child after adopting means the adoption caused it? So if Chase and I adopted a baby right now and then kept trying and got pregnant then that means that the adoption caused us to get pregnant? I don't think so!"

Jadie began pacing and Keira was shocked and concerned at how much this conversation was agitating Jadie. She did want to calm her down but also genuinely meant it when she said, "Honey, you're right. I didn't think about it like that. I don't even know where those comments came from. I guess I'd just heard about that and thought I'd share. I'm sorry that it hurt you. I certainly didn't mean to."

Jadie stopped pacing and hung her head for a moment. Keira thought her heart might break when she saw the vulnerable look on her daughter's face and the tears streaming down her face as she lifted her face.

"I know you're not trying to hurt me, momma. But this hurts." She gulped. "It hurts so so bad. I might never have a family. I might never raise kids. I may never hold a child of my own. My greatest dream in my mind is Chase and I sitting on a porch swing as we watch our grown children and grandchildren playing in our yard. We'll have had a long and happy life together and sit holding hands and watching our family. My greatest wish is to raise my kids to live for the Lord and watch them do the same with their kids. I've always wanted to be a wife and a momma and what if I never get to? What if I leave no legacy at all? What if when you and Daddy are gone, Chase and I just grow old and then die alone? I can't imagine that future, momma, but it's one I have to wonder if I'll have."

Keira fought with everything in her not to cry, but her throat was so tight she could hardly swallow and tears were making her vision blurry.

Jadie began pacing again and raised her voice as she cried and talked at the same time. Every once in awhile she would stop and face Keira and hold her hands out to the sides, palm up as she let all of her pent up feelings out. "Do you know how it feels to watch pregnant women and know I might never get to experience that? To know I may never know what Chase and I in one little person would look like or be like? I just sit here waiting and wondering and waiting and wondering, hurt and confused and in a fog. Sometimes I feel like I've fallen into a deep hole and I have no idea how to get out. It's dark and I can't even see to know where to begin to climb out. It's a horrible feeling to have my future be a big question mark. Not just my future, but something as important as this. As having my own children. I always knew I wanted to have kids, but when I married Chase, that desire went up by one hundred times. And I just want it so bad but I don't know if I'll ever have it. The uncertainty is eating me alive! And I don't feel like I'm even a real woman."

Keira felt like she'd had a bucket of cold water thrown over her and was in the cold and had no way to recover from it. No towel to dry off with and nowhere to go inside and warm up. Hearing her daughter spill all these things was so horrible to watch. She wished she could take the pain for her. And knowing that her daughter may never get to experience that kind of love for her own child made her heart break even more. She covered her still gaping mouth as tears coursed down her cheeks and she continued to listen and try to absorb what Jadie was saying.

"I don't feel normal or whole. God made women to be able to carry babies. I was designed to do that and I can't. I'm not normal. I'm not complete. My body doesn't do what it's supposed to do . . . what it was made to do. I feel like something is wrong with me. Why can't I get pregnant? What is wrong with me?" She was nearly sobbing now as she spoke. "And to top it all off, I feel like no one understands. I don't want to tell people because it feels personal and because I feel ashamed because I can't do what it seems like nearly everyone else can. It's like I'm broken, but I don't even know what's broken or how to fix it or if I can. So I feel like I suffer alone and in silence. But then if I tell people I feel like it's opening up this vulnerable part of me that's scary to share and then they don't understand me. They have no idea what I'm going through or how this feels. How horribly it hurts. I just . . . I just . . ."

Jadie dropped to her knees and couldn't go on. She felt like an idiot for going on and on, but at the same time it felt cathartic to get it all out. She was glad she'd had this meltdown in front of her momma who knew and loved her instead of someone she didn't know as well.

Keira quickly moved to the floor and held her daughter as she sobbed. She stroked her hair and said, "I'm so so sorry, honey. It's gonna be okay. I'm so sorry for what I said. You're right that people don't understand. I'm sure you can't fully unless you've been there. I'm sorry you feel isolated by this." Jadie's heart was warmed so much that her mother understood that she felt that way. She listened intently as she continued. "You just tell me what you need from me, honey, and I'll give it. Tell me what you need me to say or not say. I don't understand and I certainly don't want to hurt you. But I'm so sorry that you and Chase are going through this. You will make an amazing mother one day and I am sure you will have your family one way or another. Mother's know these things, so just trust me on that." Jadie couldn't help but laugh slightly as she still cried. "Just keep hanging in there honey. Daddy and I will be praying for you guys. And the Lord is with you through it all. It'll be okay, you'll see. I'm so sorry, baby. I'm here for you. Shhhh."

Jadie's sobs quieted some as her mother held and reassured her. She was suddenly glad she'd told her mom what was going on. It felt wonderful to have someone know and be comforting her and knowing they would be praying.

After Jadie had calmed down, she and Keira talked for a few

more minutes about the situation and then decided to watch their movie. It made them both laugh and put their minds on other things. When the guys got home, Chase had given her a quizzical look since her eyes were red and puffy. She had shaken her head and smiled to reassure him and given him a look like "I'll tell you later." They went on to have a wonderful evening together and a lovely meal. As Jadie went to go to sleep that night, she felt happy. She also felt closer to her mom. Something she didn't even know was possible.

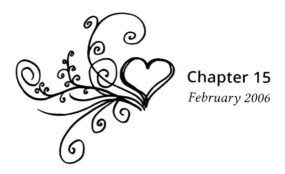

Chapter 15
February 2006

Kendra read through e-mails from her TTC group on her lunch break. She had never shared her own name or Daniel's, she always just used their initials. The day after Emma had not been feeling well and Steve had taken her to the hospital back in September, a girl named Emma had written saying she'd had a miscarriage for the fifth time. Kendra only had Emma's work e-mail and so she wasn't sure if it was the same Emma or not, but she had a feeling it was. Emma had come back to work after taking a few personal days and thanked Kendra for her help but never said what happened. Kendra was just relieved she was better. But Emma smiled less and less these days and seemed more withdrawn in herself. Emma still tried to talk to Kendra once or twice a week and Kendra had been obliging her more and more often. She didn't tell Emma anything personal, but she was civil and even tried to be nice. But secretly Kendra hoped it wasn't the same Emma on the TTC group because she had just written again last week that she'd had another miscarriage. Her sixth one and this time at eight weeks. Kendra had nearly cried reading this Emma's thoughts and feelings about losing her baby. She couldn't imagine the pain. She glanced over at Emma now and saw her sitting just slightly slumped and just staring at a sandwich and apple that were untouched on her desk. Her heart clenched and she felt a lump rise in her throat.

After observing Daniel, having several long talks with him, and a couple of brief conversations about God with Emma, Kendra had done the hardest thing she could imagine. She had humbled herself completely before the Creator of the universe and asked for His forgiveness for her sins and accepted Jesus as her personal Savior. The weight that was lifted from her shoulders and the peace she was given was indescribable. God had worked very hard on her over the months and she'd given her life to Him in January. Already the changes in her were startling even to herself and the desire to change grew by the day. She was trying to become a much more lovable and kind person. She also now realized that needing God or people or wanting them in your life was nothing to be ashamed about. She and Daniel had been meeting once a week with the Pastor of their new church as well as reading books and doing devotions together each evening after dinner. Kendra was soaking it all up like an eager sponge. There was just so much to learn, but she was determined to grow until the Lord took her home one day. Her tumultuous thoughts back in September had continued to plague her and she realized that she had allowed Satan to feed her lies to hold her back from people. Kendra supposed he knew it was easier to hold people down when they were alone. But during all of her thinking she realized that if she only let her husband and children see who she really was and was not just aloof but unkind to everyone around her, what kind of an example would that set for her children? And even if she was kind to them, what kind of mother would that make her? They would still see her act that way. It had disturbed her greatly and the Holy Spirit had used that along with her husband and Emma's testimonies to show her the truth. She had bucked against it for awhile, but finally the influences on her won out and she had difficulty in yielding, but once she did it caused great reward.

Coming out of her musing, Kendra once again glanced at

poor, sad Emma. She said a quick prayer and resolved, before she could change her mind, to initiate a conversation with Emma. She walked over to her desk and made her voice kind and said, "Hey Emma."

Emma started a bit and then looked up at her. "Oh! Hi, Kendra."

She seemed too startled to say anything else, so Kendra tried to pick up the conversation.

After a few minutes of small talk and about work, Kendra forced herself to take a deep breath and plunge ahead. Maybe by sharing she could even make a new friend.

"Emma, I've been meaning to tell you something. And I ... well, I wanted to thank you because I think God used you in helping me to see ... Well, I don't know quite how to say it, but I just wanted to tell you that I accepted Christ as my Savior last month."

Emma's eyes had grown huge at this admission and then quickly filled with tears.

"Thank you for telling me."

Before Emma could change her mind she forced herself to give Kendra a quick hug. She had no idea the wonders that did for her boss' ever-warming heart.

"I don't know what's come over me," Kendra added, trying to lighten the mood. "Must be all the hormones I'm taking."

Emma smiled and said, "Oh?"

Kendra sat on the corner of Emma's desk and smiled shyly. "Yeah, I have been going through the whole IVF process, so I'm pretty much pumped full of everything imaginable right now."

"Oh wow!" Emma said with real enthusiasm. "Congratulations! I had no idea! Where are you at in the whole process?"

"Well, right now we're in the two week wait." She covered her mouth with her hand slightly embarrassed. "Sorry, I'm used to trying to conceive 'lingo' ... we are past implantation and everything and are waiting to find out if it took."

During those sentences she'd watched Emma's face go ashen. "Emma? What is it?"

Emma tried to school her features, but it didn't work. She

slowly licked her lip and then asked, "Do you mind me asking what your husband's name is?"

Kendra felt a bit puzzled but said, "No, I don't mind. His name is Daniel. Why do you ask?"

Emma grabbed onto her desk with both hands. "Are you . . . have you . . . what I mean to say is . . . ummm . . ."

Kendra did something she'd never really done before and reached out and touched Emma's arm briefly and gave her a reassuring smile. "What is it, Emma? You can ask me."

Still wide-eyed, Emma licked her lips again and said, "Do you happen to be on a TTC group online?" and went on to say the specific name of the group.

Now Kendra's eyes grew and her face went ashen, but not for the reason that Emma thought.

"Oh, I'm so sorry for asking Kendra! That's personal and private and well . . . I apologize."

Kendra quickly shook her head. "No, it's okay . . . really! It's not that, I just . . . I am on that group. It made me realize you are . . . well the same Emma and I just feel so terrible for . . . well, for your losses."

Emma felt as though the world had just tilted a bit off it's axis. All this time she'd read update after update from "K" and never realized it was her boss. Emma had been on the group since after her first miscarriage and had the feeling when she joined "K" had been there for some time. What were the odds that they would both be members of a group that had hundreds of women on it from the entire country? She also was startled by the huge change in Kendra. Her much gentler and even shy way of opening up. And the way, if she wasn't mistaken, Kendra's eyes had even gotten slightly teary at the mention of her miscarriages.

Emma opened her mouth and closed it a few times but nothing came out as she gawked at her boss.

Finally she swallowed and allowed an almost awkward laugh to come out.

"I just can't believe it! I mean . . . what are the odds? I just . . .

it's unbelievable! What an amazing coincidence."

Emma was surprised and humbled at her boss' meek response. "Providence, really. Apparently God has been using us to help each other more than we realized."

Emma could only nod. She'd been praying for her boss and whatever was going on in her life and that God could use her while at the same time praying for "K" and her infertility issues. All along it had been the same person. And while "K"'s responses on the group had always been shorter, she had encouraged Emma several times. Amazing!

Emma had just been praying in her head that God would bring some good of all she was going through in one way or another or to use her in some way to help bring glory to Him. She had just been feeling useless. Not being able to carry babies to term made her feel less of a woman somehow at times. It was what she was designed to do and she couldn't do it. It felt as though nature itself was against her. She had just been thinking how easy it would be to let the anger she sometimes carried around in the background of her soul to come to the forefront and be mad at God. But now He had just shown her He was using her for good and she didn't even know it! Not only that, but she was just blown away by His infinite wisdom and the way He worked in her life. Silently she quickly prayed asking God to forgive her for wanting to be angry with Him and made a mental note to pray more later.

Kendra and Emma continued their conversation for several more minutes and came back around to the IVF. "How are you feeling, Kendra? From reading on the group it seems like there is so much that goes into it."

Kendra sighed and rolled her eyes slightly. "Oh, is there ever! I had been taking all kinds of injectible hormones so that they could get several good eggs. Plus I've had to do some blood work and other things along the way. Then I did a shot of HCG to cause me to ovulate. They put me under for a procedure to withdraw the eggs, then all the lab stuff took a few days, and then they did the procedure where they put the embryo's in my uterus. Now I'm taking even more hormones to make sure everything goes right." She laughed, but it didn't sound very full of mirth, but more like out of exhaustion.

Emma shook her head and her eyes were wide with wonder. She'd heard women on the group describe the process, but Emma couldn't imagine going through it personally. It just seemed kind of scary and stressful on top of having so much emotion and financial expense behind it all while hoping it had worked. "My goodness! I'm sorry it's come to that, but I'm glad you had the option."

"I know just what you mean and I'm really grateful too." She couldn't resist sighing again. "I just really hope this works."

Emma heard the deep longing in her voice and understood all that was behind the statement having been through infertility herself.

"I will be praying for you guys."

A light that Emma wasn't familiar with seeing in Kendra's eyes filled them. "Thank you. I appreciate it so much."

Kendra stood to go back to her desk since the lunch break was now nearly over. Emma gave her a lingering hug and they smiled at each other. Kendra for the millionth time this conversation, forced herself to open up one last time and share something. "You know, I feel like I've known you for years in a way. I just suddenly feel so comfortable with you."

Emma smiled and said teasingly, "Why Kendra! You have known me for years. You've known me for years twice."

They both laughed heartily and were both so excited from all they'd learned that they had a hard time settling down and getting back to work.

❤ ❤ ❤

It was Valentines Day and that meant the busiest day of the year at the flower shop Jadie worked at. Nearly all the employees of the shop were all there on the same day and at the same time.

146

That only happened a few days a year and today was one of them. Jadie found it hilarious that every year there were so many men who had put things off until the last minute and would come in looking completely stressed and frazzled, hoping they could still get something for their wives or girlfriends. Besides flowers the shop sold boxes of chocolates in various red or pink heart shaped packages, teddy bears, and other small gifts. Jadie had been working up front for a lot of the day. Putting final touches on arrangements that were requested, answering phones to take orders, working the cash register, and occasionally rushing to the back when she could to grab more flowers or work on arrangements. It could be a very stressful day, but in a way Jadie enjoyed both the distraction and the rush that the day brought. "Jadie, dear, will you run in the back and grab more roses?" Jadie noticed her boss, Fran, sounded frazzled and a bit tired.

"Sure! What color do we need this time?"

Fran handed a man his purchases and smiled and told him to have a nice day and after he walked away she paused with her hand on the counter and glanced at the ceiling for a moment.

"Umm . . . actually you better get all the colors. But we're lowest on red and white."

"Do you want me to help Susan with the arranging too?"

Fran glanced around the shop. Two men were perusing the shop and only two customers were at the registers at the moment.

"Yeah, I think you had better. Things have slowed down for the moment and I'll probably need you out front again soon, so we should take advantage of the time. Yes, please help Susan. Just get as many done as you can in the next hour and then come check with me again. If we need you before, we'll send someone back for you."

Jadie smiled. "Okay."

She didn't mind a break from working up front. She really enjoyed arranging too and at the moment, Susan was working alone again.

Jadie walked past the open area where Susan was working

and turned right down a small hallway that led to a storage room. She leaned down and pulled out more flowers from where they had them accessible and out on shelves in the hallway. There were shelves and some cupboards and counter space around the square table that Susan was working on as well. Past them and away from the actual shop was also an area with lockers for all the workers, bathrooms, and a small break room.

Once she had an armful of flowers she rushed to where Susan was and sat some on the table and some on some open counter space near them.

Susan's dark blonde hair was stuck to her face just slightly as she perspired. She looked up at Jadie with a relieved and hopeful expression. "Please tell me you are coming to help me for awhile." She then blew her breath out to blow some stray hairs out of her eyes.

Jadie smiled at her. "Yep! Sure am! Fran says I can stay and help for an hour unless they need me before."

Susan gave an exaggerated sigh. "Thank heavens!"

Jadie just laughed and they set to work. They talked for a time and then grew pre-occupied with their work and were quiet. Jadie focused as they made a couple of arrangements of soft pink and white roses with some other small additions in a thin vase with a thick, soft pink ribbon tied around the vase. She also started a couple arrangements that were similar, but also included red roses.

Jadie allowed her mind to wander as she worked and thought back to that morning with a smile. She had gotten to work early since Fran opened a couple of hours early on Valentines Day in case someone wanted to pick something up before work. So Jadie had been up and ready and to the shop by five thirty a.m. since they were opening at six. Chase had been able to get some overtime this week since they were working a big job so Jadie only woke him up briefly to give him a kiss and tell him good-bye before leaving. She wanted him to get his rest as he had been working a lot of hours. But when she arrived at work and went to her locker there was a heart shaped card taped to the front. She had smiled and read his sweet note and then opened her locker to find flowers, some of her favorite candy that he had put into a jar and curled ribbon and put on it, and a card.

He was such a sweet man. So thoughtful. Sometimes they fought a little easier than they used to on days where they were both stressed out, but most of the time she felt like they were much closer for all they'd been through with waiting to have a baby.

The scent of roses and baby's breath assailed Jadie's senses. She never tired of the smell of flowers no matter how much she worked with them. She breathed in deeply and savored the smell. They may be going through a hard time, but there were so many things she enjoyed about life. She tried to focus on those things more and be grateful for what she had. Amy had taught her a lot about that since she'd known her and she was grateful for the reminder.

Fran's husband had arrived at the shop at five p.m. to help and Fran had let Jadie go home. They were quite busy again but wouldn't be closing until seven and Fran didn't want Jadie staying that late since she was one of the first employees to arrive that day. Jadie slumped against the door for a moment and breathed out with relief when she got home. Chase was working late and wouldn't be home for another hour. Jadie went into their bedroom to change and make her hair look presentable before she and Chase went out to dinner. While she was picking out clothes, trying to find random things, picking up their bedroom some, and once she got her curling iron heating up, she decided to check the mail from her group. There were only a few, but one of them stood out to her. She finished getting changed and applied her makeup and then read it again with interest. Someone who was fairly new the group was talking about something called luteal phase defect. Jadie had never heard of that before and read the woman's description of it with interest. She had also shared links to a couple of her charts to illustrate what she was talking about.

The thing that was interesting to Jadie was that the woman's cycle was regular and was usually between twenty-eight to thirty days. She also got positive OPK's, so everything seemed normal. But she ovulated late in her cycle making her luteal phase, the time between ovulation and when she started her period again, quite short. She explained how she had been to a fertility specialist for it and they had confirmed with tests that she had low progesterone. They were going to be putting her on an oral supplement to help her progesterone levels. Jadie had at first wondered what the problem was since she ovulated. But the woman had explained that with LPD (that was the abbreviation she gave for it), since enough progesterone was not being produced, the uterus was not being prepared the way it should be, so even if conception occurred her body would just start her period anyways causing her to have an early miscarriage. Light bulbs were going off in Jadie's mind and she was so curious. She wondered if maybe there was a connection between this woman's problem and her own. She too had a normal cycle, but tended to ovulate late. Jadie nearly had to pry her eyes from the screen and then went to do her hair all the while contemplating what she had learned.

Once she was completely ready to go and since she still had fifteen minutes to spare, she started perusing everything she had written down about her cycles. She pulled out her notes and went through all the cycles where she had used OPK's and kept track of her cycle days. She held some small pieces of paper in her lap and got out a notebook and pen. She quickly googled how to count the luteal phase and found it started the day after ovulation up until the day before your next period began. Jadie began to look at her papers and count quietly aloud and then say the numbers as she wrote them down for each cycle.

"Let's see … this month it was … ok … four, five, six, seven … Okay, eight days total for that one. Nine days. Eight days."

By the time she was done she glanced at the clock and Chase would be home any second.

She suddenly felt warm and in a way anxious. *What if this*

is it? What if this is why we haven't gotten pregnant for the past fifteen months? She felt the color drain from her face for a moment and spoke quietly and aloud to herself. "Wait. No, we would have been getting pregnant. Just losing the . . ." She couldn't finish. It was too hard a possibility to even consider right now. Not until she was sure.

She heard the front door and glanced up. She went out to meet Chase by the door. He flashed her a smile even though she could tell he was tired. He was really dirty as well. He was already stripping his coat and had his gloves off. "Hey honey! Sorry I'm a few minutes late."

She felt a little dazed. "That's okay."

He bent down slightly to catch her eye. "You okay? You look so serious. Long day?"

She realized she hadn't smiled and probably did look very solemn. She smiled just slightly. "Yes, it was a long day. But more than that." She let her voice trail off and was staring again.

He took her hand and she came to and looked at him again. "What? What is it?"

"I just . . . I think I might know why it's not been working. Maybe."

He knew what she was talking about without her having to specify. "Really? Why?"

She followed him into their bedroom while he got out of his dirty work clothes and she stood in the bathroom while he took his shower and filled him in on what she had read. She finished with, "I'll have to do some more research. I had never heard of this before today."

He raised his voice just slightly to be heard above the sound of the water. "Do you think there is a way to tell without going to the doctor though?"

"I'm not sure. I want to find out. I'm sure we'd have to go to the Doctor to confirm it and if we wanted the medicine to treat it obviously."

"Well, if that is it, at least it's treatable." he said with optimism.

Still solemn and staring into space a lot as she processed, Jadie gave a quick nod forgetting that he couldn't see her. "Yeah, that is really good."

A few minutes later Chase was dressed and putting on cologne and the finishing touches. He glanced at Jadie. "Perk up, will you? If this is it, that's good news! At least we know it's something that's easy to fix."

"Yeah, that's what Sharon said."

"Sharon?"

"The lady who posted about it."

"Ahh. Well yeah, it would be good to know it's an easy fix."

Jadie glanced at him and his eyes were still on the mirror. "Yes, but it also means there is something to fix which isn't a nice realization. I was still hoping maybe nothing was wrong."

Chase stopped what he was doing and turned towards her for a moment. "You're right honey, I know that's not what we wanted." He sighed and thought for a moment. "But it has been a year and a few months. I guess we had a good idea something was wrong. It would just be nice to find out this easily and hopefully fix it just as easily."

"I know. That is good. But . . . but . . ."

He touched her arm gently. "What honey?"

She licked her lips. "Well, if that is what I do have, that means that . . . that we could have been getting pregnant and losing . . . losing the . . ."

She let her voice trail off and looked up at him with pained eyes. She saw the realization dawn there. He put both hands on each of her arms and said in a very sensitive tone, "We could have been losing babies."

She just nodded. He pulled her into a hug. She saw the sadness on his face too and while she didn't like that they were facing this possibility, she was glad to know he understood and felt the same way as her about it all.

He pulled back and looked at her and smiled. "I didn't have a chance to tell you how beautiful you look tonight."

She blushed just slightly like she always did when he said that and she smiled a little.

"Thank you. You look really nice too."

He took hold of her arms again. "Listen honey. I know this is a lot for us to take in. But we don't know for sure yet. Do your research tomorrow. Then we'll talk about where we should go from there. But let's go out to dinner and enjoy our Valentines Day, okay?"

She took a deep breath and smiled at him. "Yeah. You're right and I would like that."

They held hands and walked towards the front door. It was the beginning of a wonderful evening. To Jadie's surprise, she only thought of it briefly and in passing throughout the evening and just had a great time with her husband.

The next day Jadie had to work again, but she still got home before Chase. She had really enjoyed their evening the night before, but today she had been anxious to get home and look up more about luteal phase defect. So as soon as she got home she did just that. She researched it quite a bit and learned more about it in general and also that doctors seemed to agree that a fourteen day luteal phase was ideal, twelve was pretty good, but ten was not good and anything from that point and lower was considered an automatic luteal phase defect diagnosis. Jadie glanced at the numbers she had written down the day before. Her luteal phase was usually eight or nine days but most often eight. From her research, that definitely signaled a problem.

When Chase got home she relayed all of this to him and also showed him some things she had found. They then moved to the couch in the living room and talked about it some more.

"So, what do you think we should do then?" Chase asked after they'd been quiet for a moment.

"Well, I think I should start charting. I'd been avoiding it because I didn't want to focus on that every day and it seems really complicated, but I think it would be good to do so we can show a doctor what's going on with my body. It would also show hopefully that my temps confirm what the OPK's are saying about when I ovulate."

Chase shook his head slightly. "I still think it's crazy that you can enter your temperatures into that website and it will show a pattern to show when you ovulate."

"Yeah, it's pretty amazing. So what do you think about going to the doctor?"

"Well, it seems pretty sure that you have this thing. But to confirm it and get help for it, we do need to see a doctor. I hate to wait, but my job is just starting to pick up. We should be caught up and in a more comfortable position financially soon. What do you think?"

"Well, from what I've heard fertility specialists often like you to chart for three months so they can see a pattern with your body. What if we stop trying for the next three months so that we don't have to worry about getting pregnant and miscarrying and I'll chart during that time. I can call and get a referral from my doctor and it usually takes awhile to get into a fertility specialist, so hopefully by the time three months is up we'd have an appointment and be ready financially to go as well."

Chase thought for a moment. "That sounds like it will all work out really well. It's hard to wait when we have a good idea what's going on, but I think it would be best if we did it this way for all the reasons you mentioned."

"Yeah, it will be hard to wait. But I think it'll save time to already have charted by the time we go to the specialist and if we have to wait anyways to get in and financially, it just makes sense to do it that way. It will be worth it if in a few months we can be on our way to solving the problem."

Chase agreed. "So do you think we should go right to a specialist and not your regular doctor then?"

She shrugged. "I think it would be best. If I had cancer I'd go straight to an oncologist because that's their specialty. They know a lot more about it. I'd just feel more comfortable going to someone that specializes in that area. It just seems like they'll know more about it and how to handle it better."

"Makes sense to me. Well, we have a plan. It feels good to know where we're going. It just stinks that it involves more waiting."

"It does, but it feels really good to have a plan. It's tough not knowing what to do about something. At least it seems like we have found out at least part of what could be wrong and knowing how we're going to go about fixing it. It's nice to not have everything out there," she gestured with her hand out in front of her, "just all question marks."

"Yeah, the uncertainty is terrible. So it is nice to have something solid to go on."

Jadie agreed with him. In a way she already felt so much better. But facing going to a specialist and potentially having to do expensive and uncomfortable tests wasn't fun to think about either. She comforted herself that at least soon they'd be on their way to answers and hopefully a baby as a result.

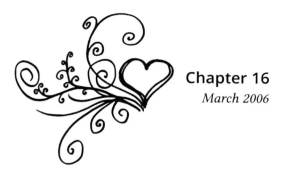

Chapter 16
March 2006

Amy lay still on the table in the same building Dr. Moyer's office was in. She had been told to relax for fifteen minutes before she could get up, get dressed, and go home. She had just had her second IUI procedure done. Now it was time to wait for a couple of weeks and come back and have a test to see if it worked. More waiting. And never had there been more pressure as she knew this was probably she and Jake's last attempt at a biological child.

She squeezed her eyes shut and prayed that God would give her strength to wait in the coming weeks and to accept whatever the outcome was.

There used to be a time where Amy may have not known entirely how she felt about someone having medical intervention to have children. But after experiencing infertility herself, she now felt it was a very personal decision and one each couple had to make for themselves. From being on her group, she knew nearly everyone else she knew with infertility felt the same way and were all supportive of each other's decisions. There were so many options now. Natural or treatment-wise, things you could do at home, vitamins to take to try to help, medications and procedures depending on if you went to a specialist, and on and on it went. She understood completely everyone who went either direction, of not trying anything to help or going all the way through the process and to IVF, sometimes even multiple times. Amy believed that things could go wrong with someone's body in many ways on this earth and that as humans we are blessed to have doctors and treatments to help and she saw infertility as no different. Whether someone used treatment or not, God was the only Creator of life.

She sighed and draped her forearm over her forehead. Only a few more minutes and she could get out of the uncomfortable gown and go home. She and Jake both disliked going to the doctor for any reason quite a bit and so something this personal definitely made them both uncomfortable. But it was worth it to have a shot at a biological child.

Since Amy and Jake's families had known for awhile now about their infertility, they had somewhat allowed the news to spread and occasionally shared about it with others. The "when are you going to have kids?" question was nearly driving them as mad as the comments when they did choose to share. So they decided to just put it out there and at least people from church could be praying for them. You could never have too much prayer! They had received a lot of hurtful comments, but some people just didn't know what to say and offered to pray which was both nice and comforting. Amy realized through sharing it with more people just how little it was understood. They had even had a couple people tell them they were going through the same thing, but just hadn't shared. Amy and Jake both had be-friended two couples at church that they didn't know about before and it had been a great help to them all. Amy was shocked though at how many people told them that maybe that was God's will for them to be childless and they should just adopt. Adoption was talked about, and even pushed, a lot it seemed. Amy and Jake both felt adoption was wonderful, but sometimes it seemed like people wanted to make them feel guilty for wanting a child of their own or that they didn't deserve the opportunity to try. It was something that had surprised her, but when she shared about it on her group, she found other women who had people tell them the same things and had gotten the same impression. It was just one more way to make people with infertility not want to share their pain and one more way for them to feel isolated. Amy felt like she and Jake had just as much of a right to want biological children as anyone else. There was nothing wrong with wanting to have a child of their own even though they were also pursuing adoption. She also wondered if people realized how much emotional stress and financial strain adoption could cause as well. For people with infertility, any road chosen to the children of their dreams was not an easy one.

Being where she was, it also caused her to reflect back on how when she had joined her group, she knew nothing about all the options and treatments available. While she had heard of IVF especially and rarely IUI, she didn't really understand what all was involved. Even once she had learned the difference between the two and what all went into it, experiencing it for herself was another thing entirely. Some women had terrible experiences just with Clomid or other drugs used to help conceive, but the IUI and IVF processes involved a lot of appointments, hormones, and expense to accomplish the procedure. IUI was cheaper, but also had a lower success rate. She'd done a lot of research and while it could be affected by different circumstances unique to each couple (like a man's sperm count for instance), it seemed like 15-25% was an average success rate. Which was why many people had to attempt it multiple times or move onto IVF if it didn't work and they wanted to keep trying. She thought back to how she had gone through this whole process now a second time and she was relieved it was over, even if she was nervous that maybe it wouldn't work. She wasn't a weak woman, but it certainly wasn't enjoyable. She personally had done blood work and urine samples towards the beginning of her cycle as well as an ultrasound to look at her uterus, follicles, and other reproductive organs; followed by taking injections (she knew some women on her group who had taken pills instead) to help her follicles grow.

She had learned that the follicles were the things where the eggs grew inside the ovaries and that they needed to grow to make a mature egg. The follicles were measured at least a couple of times during the cycle to make sure they were growing to the proper size. Dr. Moyer wanted them somewhere in the high teens to the low twenties in millimeters for them to be considered the right size. She had heard of some poor women getting over-stimulated from the hormones, which could be very painful, and they were unable to do the procedure and had to start all over again later. Other women's follicles didn't grow properly even with the hormones and they too had to scrap their procedures. Amy's heart went out to them even more now that she understood how difficult it could all be on top of already sensitive emotions. Both times in her case the follicles had grown properly and then she was given what was called a "trigger shot" of HCG which caused her to ovulate. Within a short time period of that happening, they then came into the office and Jake gave a sperm sample which was then "washed" so it was just pure and good sperm to increase the chance of a good result. Then it was placed directly into Amy's uterus in a procedure that took only a few minutes and wasn't too terribly uncomfortable. Amy knew from being on her group that there were some variations to the process depending on the fertility problems each couple had. But that's what it was like for her and Jake. She was thankful that the procedure had worked so well for them both times. Now if it would just work entirely and they could be pregnant.

At this point if they got pregnant Amy would hardly know what to think! It would feel like a dream and would be hard to take in. For now, she tried to just find that tiny little line of having hope and faith, but not having her hopes up. She could pray however, so she did again, asking God to help it to work for them this time and again that she and Jake would accept whatever outcome came of it. She did this quietly until the nurse came in and told her she could get dressed and go home. As she dressed, she prayed one more time for peace to wait over the next couple of weeks. She knew they were going to feel like the longest of her life.

♥ ♥ ♥

The rhythmic clickity clack of the shopping cart as it glided across the floor of the grocery store nearly put Jadie into a trance. She was watching where she was going, but nothing seemed to be registering. Chase reached over and gently covered her right hand with his own.

"Honey, are you alright? You seem a bit distracted."

Jadie stopped pushing the shopping cart and looked up at her husband's handsome face. How she loved that man. He was so loving and always so concerned about her. She gave him a sweet smile.

"I'm fine. I suppose I am distracted though." She began to push the cart again and looked ahead. She let out a sigh and then continued. "Jake and Amy had their second IUI attempt today and it's just been on my mind."

Chase gently smacked his palm against his forehead and leaned back slightly and then continued walking. "Oh yeah! I had forgotten about that. You told me yesterday and I even prayed for them this morning, but it slipped my mind again. You know me." He playfully wiggled his eyebrows at her.

She laughed. "Indeed I do. Anyways, I just feel so bad for all they've had to go through and I'm just really hoping this is it for them."

Chase nodded and turned serious. "I do too. I feel like I know them so well through you and I just really feel for them."

Jadie smiled inwardly. She loved how he could go from that twinkly-eyed almost boyish guy to serious and concerned in just a few seconds. He was serious when he needed to be and was very level headed. Yet his playful side came out daily and he was also so easy to smile and laugh. She thought that made the perfect combo.

Chase realized Jadie hadn't replied and said, "Did I lose you again?"

She shook her head and smiled. "No. I was just thinking about what a wonderful man you are."

A huge grin slowly spread across his face and that visible twinkle came into his eye that she was so familiar with. "You're just now figuring that out?"

She rolled her eyes, grinned, and playfully pushed him with her elbow. "Listen to you!"

He grinned at her for a few more seconds and then watched ahead of him again. "Hey, come down this aisle, will you? I think something I need is down here."

Jadie turned the cart and swung into the aisle he'd mentioned. Just then a pregnant woman walked by holding her husband's hand. They were smiling at each other and the husband had a couple of tiny blue outfits tucked under his arm.

As Chase was examining a couple of things he needed to fill in some gaps in his tool box he said, "We need to remember to pray for Jake and Amy before we go to bed tonight."

"Absolutely."

Jadie's heart went out to her friend. At the moment it also clenched in the all-too-familiar pain it felt whenever she saw someone who was pregnant. *Does she realize what she has? How lucky and blessed she is? How many of us are silently suffering and want that so badly?* She chastised herself. Amy was always reminding her to be thankful for what she had . . . for what God had given her. Jadie tried to remind herself of that often. She didn't want to envy people she didn't even know. It was just hard sometimes to watch that and yearn so badly for it that she could feel a physical ache inside. She couldn't help but wonder too what it would be like to be pregnant. To have your own sweet little baby growing and developing inside of you. To feel their sweet kicks every day and know that they could hear your voice. *What does it feel like?* The question came to her every time she witnessed it. She wanted so badly to experience it for herself and to feel what it was like.

She shook her head hoping to dispel the thoughts from her

mind. Many times a day she thought about her infertility and her longing to have a child. She tried to not let it consume her as it seemed it was often trying to do, but that didn't mean that it wasn't on her heart daily and that it didn't hurt.

Chase tossed a couple things into the cart they needed and was ready to keep moving, so Jadie blew out her breath as she began to push the cart again and hoped that she could put it all from her mind for now.

She and Chase got caught up talking about every day things when it seemed like every pregnant woman on the planet had also decided to shop this very night. Jadie felt frustrated that she couldn't seem to ever escape her feelings from infertility. Just when she'd gotten distracted by talking to Chase, she began to notice all these pregnant women shopping. There were even two friends who couldn't be very far apart in how far along they were laughing together as they shopped. She had turned and was looking for something on the shelf when a girl who was probably sixteen years old at most stepped near her to get something. Jadie glanced at her and smiled and then noticed her baby bump. She forced her eyes back to the shelf and tried to look normal as she searched for what she needed. She didn't want the girl to feel judged by her. Jadie was feeling things for an entirely different reason. Once the girl went on her way, her ever-observant Chase asked her what was wrong.

"Oh, just that girl. She couldn't have been a day over sixteen. Even she is pregnant! Why do teenage girls who aren't ready to be parents get pregnant and people like us who are stable and married can't? It just makes no sense!"

Chase listened with a concerned face and then replied, "It does seem unfair in a way. I'm not gonna lie, that can be very hard to see when we're in the situation we're in."

Jadie felt her frustration mounting. "Are we not going to be good parents? Are we being punished for something?" She slammed something into the cart and Chase winced a little.

"I have had feelings like that too, but I don't think that's the case. Maybe God is just trying to teach us something? I really don't understand it, honey." Jadie had to look away from her husband's too somber face.

She tried to swallow the near bitterness she felt rising up in her throat. Thoughts like *"it's not fair"* and *"why them and not me?"* assuaged her. She felt her shoulders droop and sighed. *Lord, please help me in this near constant battle. I am trying to trust Your will in all this. Help my negativity and lack of faith.* She didn't even get a chance to feel better from her prayer before she got slammed with another remark from an almost audible voice in her head. *"If you were a good Christian you would trust God more. Maybe you should just rely on yourself instead of Him through this. After all, He could give you a baby but is deliberately choosing not to."* Jadie physically shook her head to try to dispel the thoughts. She and Amy had talked recently about how Satan tried to put thoughts in their minds. They were always negative, against God, something to beat themselves up with, or something similar. They had both come to the conclusion that they really had to be on their guard against things like that and fight against it. Jadie squared her shoulders and held herself up high. *Absolutely not! I will not give into those thoughts! Lord, thank you for all You have given me. I'm sorry I forget so often how much you have blessed me with and too often long for other things. I don't deserve anything I have and it's all a blessing from You. Chase, my family, our lovely little home, my job, and on and on it goes. I even get to spend eternity with You and that's more than enough! I know you're not doing this to hurt us, it's just hard sometimes. Help me to fight against Satan's lies and live in Your truth. Help me to remember that we live in a fallen world by our own doing and that things with our bodies just don't always work right in one way or another. Be with Jake, Amy, Chase and I, and anyone else who's struggling to have a baby. Help them to feel Your presence and I pray that You would give us our miracles in Your timing and in Your way. Amen.*

She allowed herself a few more minutes to think and then shared with Chase what she'd been thinking and had prayed.

He smiled at her. "I was doing a little praying of my own. It really can be hard to not be jealous of other people and to not be negative."

Jadie nodded. "It sure can! I remind myself so often that God's not doing this to hurt us."

Chase inhaled deeply. "You have told me that before and I've had to remind myself of that as well. I'm sure He'll bring good out of this somehow."

Jadie smiled. "I sure hope so."

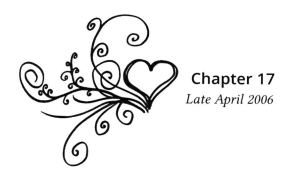

Chapter 17
Late April 2006

Birds chirped and the sun shone down on Chase and Jadie as they walked hand in hand towards the doctor's office. It was a beautiful day out and Jadie hoped it was a good sign towards what they were about to do. She felt a bit nervous, but very excited too. She had been anxiously anticipating this appointment ever since she made it over two and a half months ago. There was a fertility specialist in this building and all she'd had to do was call and get a referral from her regular physician to be able to get an appointment with her. The breeze gently blew the loose strands of Jadie's hair around her face and she gently tucked them behind her ears. She smiled at Chase who gave her hand a gentle squeeze. For so long it felt like she had been in a thick fog of uncertainty and today she hoped to get some of that cloud lifted.

Jadie was glad that once she'd given the nurse her name and appointment time they didn't have to wait long. She wrung her hands a bit in anticipation until a nurse came out and called their names. They followed her through a series of hallways and then entered a room. She and Chase talked quietly until the Doctor entered the room a short time later.

She had red hair that was all one length and came to about her shoulders, was tall and thin, and had a lovely smile which she flashed them as soon as she walked into the room. She had a very open and warm manner and Jadie liked her instantly. She introduced herself to them and shook each of their hands. She started off making a joke which put Jadie and Chase even more at ease. "You've probably noticed my bright red hair and are wondering how someone who is as pale as me possibly has the last name of 'Sanchez'." Jadie and Chase smiled, but didn't say anything. Honestly Jadie hadn't even noticed the irony. "Well, Sanchez is my married name, so that's why the Latino name with the red hair." They all shared a laugh and then the Dr. began asking some questions.

Not long into the conversation Jadie handed her the charts she had printed out. February's chart wasn't complete since she started partway through a cycle, but it still showed when she ovulated. She also gave her March's chart and April's which had just finished. All three charts showed her luteal phase at just eight days. Dr. Sanchez was very pleased Jadie had brought them and they discussed them along with luteal phase defect for awhile.

Once Dr. Sanchez had asked and gotten answered many questions about their TTC up to that point, about their financial position, and plans for the future of TTC and how they wanted to proceed, she thought for a moment. Jadie sat on the edge of her seat and felt like an eternity had passed before the Dr. said thoughtfully, "Well, normally I would do a couple of tests to confirm the luteal phase defect. But you guys have already been trying for quite awhile and I hate to put you through the cost and experience of the tests." She made a quirking noise with her mouth and she looked over Jadie's charts again. "You know what? This is what I'm going to do. I'm going to give you a prescription for four months." Jadie's heart instantly soared and she continued to listen intently. "It's for an oral pill called prometrium. It's bio-identical to the progesterone your body is supposed to make. You will start taking it the day after ovulation and for fourteen days after even if your period arrives. We want to make absolutely certain you're not pregnant before you stop taking it. At that point, you'll take a pregnancy test. If it's negative, you can stop taking the prometrium for that cycle. If it's positive, you'll continue to take it to support the pregnancy. But I don't want to give you a long time's supply of this in case there is something else going on. I do know you have the luteal phase defect without doing any other tests, otherwise there is no way your luteal phase would be that short. Nothing else could be causing that. But, there is still the possibility there may be other factors hindering you from achieving pregnancy. So I'm going to do something I rarely do, and that's to let you try the prescription for four months. If you don't get pregnant within that time, I want you to come back for more tests. At that time we would get a sperm analysis set up for Chase and I will want to do blood work on you Jadie and also check to see if your tubes are clear. Then we will go from there as needed at that time. Do either of you have any questions?"

They each had a few and her answers were kind and detailed.

After talking a bit more with Dr. Sanchez, they all stood and both Chase and Jadie thanked her. "We really appreciate it!" Chase added. "It'll be great to actually be able to try something and see if it works and not have to wait on getting test results."

"You're welcome. But be sure to make an appointment right away if you don't get pregnant within that time. I usually have a waiting list." She turned towards Jadie. "When you go to pay Jadie, I'd also like you to make an appointment to have a physical with me. When you're here I'm also going to have you give a basic blood and urine sample."

"Okay, I will." Jadie could hardly keep the smile from her face.

"And be sure to keep charting as well Jadie. I want to see how you respond to the prometrium, how it effects your luteal phase, when you're ovulating, your symptoms, and so on."

"Alright, I'll do that. Thanks again, Dr. Sanchez."

"You're very welcome. Well it was nice to meet you both," she shook their hands again, "and I'll see you soon Jadie." With that, she closed the door and was gone.

Chase and Jadie grinned at each other and then hugged. They gathered their things and in no time were headed back out to the car. They talked all the way home about how great the appointment had gone and how Jadie couldn't wait to get going on this first cycle of using the medicine.

"If this is all that's wrong, we could finally be pregnant really soon!" She said excitedly. "This would just make so much sense. Why I felt like I've been pregnant before, why it hasn't been working ..." Her voice trailed off for a moment and had grown more serious. "Maybe we can get pregnant on our own; we just couldn't keep the baby. Now, we'll be able to!" Chase reached over and took her hand.

"I'm sad that we've more than likely lost babies like Dr. Sanchez thinks we have, but I am glad we know now and how to prevent it from happening."

"Me too." Jadie added fervently.

They were quiet for a moment and then Jadie smiled again and was nearly giddy as she said, "I can't wait to call Amy when we get home!"

♥ ♥ ♥

Amy and Jake held hands as they waited for Dr. Moyer to enter the room that they were waiting in at their doctor's office. Today they found out if their second IUI attempt worked. Amy felt her palms growing sweaty. She tried to take deep breaths to calm herself down. It was so difficult to not be nervous! So much rested on this news. She and Jake had decided that this was probably their last attempt at having a baby on their own. Right now it felt unbearable to consider they may never have biological children. She wanted so badly for this to work! She hoped Dr. Moyer wouldn't make them wait long.

She glanced over at Jake and he stared unblinking at the wall. She could tell by the hardened look on his handsome face that he was very worried. She had a bad feeling in the pit of her stomach. She squeezed her eyes shut and prayed, *Dear God, please help us to accept whatever news it is we're about to get. Help us to know what to do. Please, just comfort us in this time.*

She glanced at Jake again and tried to catch his eye. Once he was looking at her she gave him the best smile she could muster, which didn't even end up showing her teeth. He sighed and relaxed some and gave her a tiny smile in return. She was just about to say something when the door opened.

They both jerked their gaze to the door and Dr. Moyer had her back to them as she closed the door behind her. Amy's heart slammed into an irregular rhythm as she waited for her to turn around. When she did, her face looked grim although it held a polite smile. Amy's heart nearly sank to her feet. She tried to keep her hopes up, but she felt she already knew the news was not good.

Dr. Moyer quickly shook their hands, took a seat, and was quick in delivering what she had to say. "I'm very sorry to tell you that the procedure, once again, did not take this time."

Amy felt like someone had dumped a cold bucket of water over her head and slugged her in the stomach all at the same time. She learched forward and gasped in a breath as she realized she hadn't taken one in . . . well, she didn't know how long. Jake's mouth was hanging open from the news, but he instantly grabbed hold of Amy's arms and held her upright and asked if she was alright. Dr. Moyer had also started to stand and was reaching towards Amy, but sat back down when she saw Jake had stabilized her.

"I'm so sorry, Amy. Are you alright?"

Amy took a couple of quick breaths and nodded. "I think so. I'm just shocked and . . . very disappointed." She covered her eyes with one of her hands and was very surprised herself as a couple of tears came out. She was a very private person and hated that she kept crying in front of people.

Dr. Moyer reached out and touched her knee. "I know it's very difficult. You guys have been through a lot and this was not the news I wanted to give you today."

Amy nodded and forced herself to stop crying. She removed her hand and looked at her lap and tried to find something to study to keep her tears at bay.

Jake had his arm around her and gently rubbed her arm.

After another moment of silence Dr. Moyer said, "Well, we still have some options. With you having PCOS, Amy, I'd only suggest doing IUI one more time at the most if you guys really wanted to try that again. Or we can go right for IVF this time or do that if another IUI round fails."

Amy and Jake both began to shake their heads at the same time. They looked at each other and the pain in Amy's eyes was too much for Jake and he forced his gaze back to the Doctor.

He cleared his throat and then said, "I think we need some time to talk things over and decide what we want to do. We weren't sure we wanted to do any more procedures after this one."

Dr. Moyer looked very sad but nodded. "I understand. You had expressed to me that you may not want to attempt again after this cycle. You guys talk things over and just call and leave a message for me with what you decide. If you decide not to proceed with anything else here, then I wish you all the best."

Jake nodded and Amy continued to stare at her lap and seemed in a daze. Dr. Moyer rose, so Jake stood and helped Amy do the same. To his surprise, she hugged them both and gave them another sad smile before leaving the room.

Jake looked at his wife's stricken face. He rubbed her arms gently. "Come on, honey. Let's get you home."

On the ride home, tears would occasionally slide down her face, but she never said anything. Jake understood she needed time to process. He didn't mind having some time to himself to think either. It was a very harsh blow for sure. He knew how he felt already about where they should go from here, but he wanted to be careful about when and how he told Amy. He also wanted to hear her point of view before anything final was decided.

Jake knew this was a day he and Amy would probably never forget, regardless of what was decided. He was certain it was one of the worst days of his life, and from looking at Amy, he knew the same was true of her.

♥ ♥ ♥

Beautiful colors streaked the sky and painted a beautiful picture across the Wyoming landscape as Jake and Amy walked to their door that evening. Amy felt like it was such a stark opposite of what she felt like inside. At the same time, it felt like the sky was reflecting what she was going through: The closing of a big chapter in her life. But it was good for her to see that there was still beauty and light in the world, even if her heart felt the darkest it ever had.

Jake tossed his keys on the side table when they had walked in the door and Amy jumped. Jake flipped some lights on and Amy noticed the light on the answering machine was blinking. She pressed the button and Jadie's animated and excited voice rang through their kitchen. "Hey Amy! It's Jadie! Our appointment today went fantastic! I can't wait to tell you all about it. I'm hoping to hear awesome news from you guys too. I'm assuming you'll be home from your appointment soon." Resentment rose up in Amy for just the slightest moment and then quickly died with her friends next words which were said in a more serious tone. "I have been praying just as hard, if not harder, for you guys all day as I have been for us. I really hope it worked this time. Call me when you can. Love you! Bye."

Jadie was such a precious friend. For a moment she had been jealous that her friend must have received good news. But then she remembered how much she cared about Jadie and she would always wish her the best even if things weren't working out for her. She also remembered that sometimes just getting answers was good news; it didn't necessarily mean it was great news. She knew that if the Doctor confirmed that Jadie had luteal phase defect, that would mean she and Chase had probably lost babies and that was nothing to celebrate. She did want to talk to her friend now more than ever, but she needed to talk to her husband first.

She and Jake wordlessly moved into the living room and talked about how they were feeling for awhile. It was a very somber conversation. Amy looked up at Jake and said, "It's over, isn't it?" and then looked back to her lap.

Jake sighed and considered how to answer. "I feel like this part of our journey is over, but I want to know how you feel, too, Amy. We both need to be one hundred and ten percent sure."

A few tears slid out as Amy looked at her husband again. She felt like her heart was broken in two. "Well, we've prayed about it a lot together and separately, and deep down, yeah . . . I feel like that was our last shot and it's time to be done. We tried quite a bit and I just feel like maybe this isn't God's will for us. I'm glad we tried, but I think . . . I think . . ."

Her tears overtook her then and Jake leaned forward and pulled her into his arms. She snuggled against her husband's chest and released all the emotion of everything she was feeling. She let her tears flow and she sobbed harder than she ever had in her life.

Jake just stroked her hair and back and held her, wishing he could do something to take away her pain. At the same time, he'd never felt so much pain in his life. At least they were not alone and their hearts completely understood one another's.

He knew from multiple conversations they'd had that neither of them blamed themselves, each other, or God even though they'd been tempted to do some of those things along the way. It just wasn't meant to be for them. It was over. And even though he felt like they'd made the right decision for their family, it didn't mean that it didn't hurt. He knew they would need time to mourn the fact that they would never have children of their own.

Suddenly his face wrinkled uncontrollably and tears quickly slid down his cheeks. All his dreams of what their children would look like, be like . . . all of it dissipated right in front of him. He leaned his head against Amy's as silent sobs racked his body.

Amy wrapped her arms more tightly around Jake and they held onto each other for dear life. They would never have biological children, but they had God and they had each other. That may be all they ever had. But the pain of what was missing, for right now, seemed overwhelming.

A couple of hours later, after darkness had long overtaken the beautiful sunset from earlier, Amy dialed her friends' number. She already felt calmer and at peace. The pain was still very fresh, but God's comfort was always there.

Jadie picked up after only a couple of rings. After greeting each other, Amy insisted Jadie share her news first. Finally, Jadie gave in.

She shared all about the appointment and how Dr. Sanchez had given them a prescription to try for four months. Amy knew all they'd been through and she was so glad for them that they had an answer and also were finally able to try something knowing it might actually work. Hope swelled in her chest for her friend and she genuinely was able to be happy as she talked to her friend.

Finally Jadie said, "Alright, Amy. Please tell me." Although her voice sounded somber, Jadie hoped beyond hope that Amy was just saving the best news for last. She also knew how unselfish Amy was and worried she wanted to let Jadie have her happy moment first. Her heart beat fast and she waited for Amy to answer her. The silence on the line felt deafening.

Amy sighed and said, "It didn't work, Jadie. Jake and I have talked about it, and we've decided to be done. It's over."

Jadie was amazed, but not surprised, at her friends' practical tone. But she knew Amy well enough by now to hear some of the pain in her voice.

She gasped and her words came out a hushed whisper, "Oh, Amy! No!"

Amy choked up instantly but forced herself to say, "It's okay, Jadie. Or at least it will be."

Tears slid down Jadie's cheeks. "I am so so sorry Amy. No one deserves a baby more than you."

Amy laughed despite her tears. "Oh, I don't know about that. But thank you."

Jadie could barely talk past her clogged throat, but managed,

"I know you're going to be a momma someday Amy. I can feel it. It's going to happen, just you wait and see!"

"Thank you, Jadie. I really hope so."

"Are you . . . Jake, is he . . . Are you guys alright?"

"We're okay. We cried for about an hour straight. I have a horrible headache now and my eyes are all puffy. I'm sure there'll be more tears to come in the future too."

Chase saw Jadie gripping the phone with both hands and the tears running down her face. He grabbed her arm gently and his eyes gently asked the question. Jadie shook her head no. Chase dropped his arm and looked crestfallen. He motioned to her that he was going to go pray.

Jadie said, "Chase and I are so sorry and Chase is going to pray right now."

"Thank you." Amy said, meaning it with all her heart. She was very touched by both people.

Jadie started crying again, "Oh Amy, I'm just . . . I'm so . . ."

"I know." Amy said.

They both cried on the phone together and spoke no words for awhile. Neither of them needed to. It was a great loss and one they both mourned.

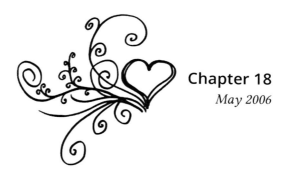

Chapter 18
May 2006

Amy sat in church surrounded by all of her family. She was holding her new niece Annie who was about two months old now. She looked down and smiled at the sweet little bundle who was glancing around this way and that as though she was trying to soak everything in. Amy glanced over at her sister Laura who had her other daughter, Suzie, snuggled in her lap. Her sister had looked great so soon after having Suzie and she seemed to have recovered even more quickly this time. She admired her sister very much as a mother. She only hoped someday she would have children to call her own. Some days she felt for sure that she would be a mother some way or another and other days she felt so hopeless. Since her and Jake's decision to no longer pursue having biological children she had been struggling more now than nearly ever since everything began over three years ago. She knew Satan was working overtime on her right now since she had been so saddened, but she had to try to fight against him discouraging her so much. She had to trust and rely on the Lord and be okay no matter the outcome. It was okay to hurt, but it was not okay for her to be in perpetual despair.

Amy was at least glad she didn't feel the gigantic hole inside of her any more when holding a baby. It still hurt, but it was better than it used to be and for that she was very grateful. Holding her niece did bring up some unpleasant thoughts and feelings, but it was also a wonderful experience and one she treasured.

Jake held her elbow to support her since she was holding the baby as they stood to sing some songs. She was grateful for his tender touch and always appreciated his thoughtfulness. He was such a wonderful man. Of course he had flaws, just like everyone else, but he was perfect for her and she knew it. She tried to remind herself of what she was always encouraging Jadie: to be thankful for what they did have instead of longing so badly for something they didn't. It wasn't bad to want to be a mother, but it was easy to become consumed by that and forget about the blessings they did have in life. Even if they never had children, she was immensely blessed to have her Savior, her soul mate, her family, and so many other things. She smiled as she sang and felt truly grateful.

She was truly happy and doing well until they began to have people share stories about their mothers. When a younger person would stand and thank their mother, Amy felt the familiar chasm inside of her along with a curiosity to know just how strong that bond and love was between a mother and her child and if she would ever experience it. She was grateful for her mother and tried to think of it from that perspective, but the whole service was about mothers today. Appropriate since it was Mother's Day after all. She just couldn't help but think how hard it was to think about and hear about all morning while she and Jake so recently had decided to stop trying to have biological children. It felt like her heart had begun to heal only a little and was now ripped open and was slowly bleeding. When the pain became too much, she passed Annie to Laura since Suzie had decided to move to her Daddy's lap, and she made her way to the ladies room to splash some water on her face. She then stayed in the foyer until the service was over. She was glad it wasn't too much longer because she didn't want people to wonder where she had gone to or why she hadn't come back in. But it was too much for her right now and Amy was fine with her decision. She felt pain from the whole situation enough and if a time arose, like now, where she could avoid some of that pain, then she was going to. It felt instinctual to protect herself and she was sure the Lord understood.

She was relieved when people filtered out of the sanctuary and no one said anything to her about it. Not much later her family all got going so they could make their lunch reservation at a restaurant about twenty minutes away. Amy was relieved to be going. Once she and Jake were seated in the car, Jake reached over and squeezed her hand. Amy raised her eyebrows momentarily and cocked her head slightly for a moment and released a long breath at the same time. Jake understood without her saying a word and gave her a reassuring smile and then released her hand and drove out of the parking lot and onto the road.

Many miles away, Jadie was trying to endure the Mother's Day service she was attending as well. The songs, people's testimonies, and the shorter sermon were all geared towards being a mother or how you felt about your mother, and so on. Jadie, like Amy, had been trying to focus on her mother instead of wondering if she would ever be a mother herself. She too found it nearly impossible to do that completely however.

She couldn't help but wonder if there were other people in the service like her who were suffering through the same thing. Sometimes she felt like people with infertility were not even on most people's radar and they didn't even consider how someone going through that may be feeling at a time like this. She tried not to think about people harshly for that though because she knew she used to never think about it either … until it happened to her. She was saddened by human's tendencies to be selfish and only think of themselves and the problems they had faced only and not what other people might be experiencing. She felt disappointed in herself for never considering people who went through something like that until she herself was going through it. *Why are we like that?* she wondered. She realized she could still be like that in some regards. Sure, she was considerate of people who went through infertility now, but only because she was amongst them. There were still things she didn't think about much that people went through and she could probably be more sensitive. Losing a spouse or having cancer were just two things that popped into her head as she glanced at some of the people in front of her in just a couple of rows.

She closed her eyes and prayed, *Dear Lord, please help me to be more thoughtful and considerate of all those around me who are going through or have been through something really tough whether I've experienced it myself or not. Help me to be more aware of what I'm saying and doing and to always be thinking of others even if I don't know what they're going through. I don't want to walk on egg shells obviously around every one, but help me to be more considerate of others while still making them feel comfortable and loved around me, Lord. Amen.*

Jadie was surprised that she went from condemning others for not considering her to realizing she was doing the same thing so quickly. She realized everyone had a tendency to do that and that she was not innocent in that area by any means. But she was aware now and wanted to do better.

Now to just try to make it through the rest of the service without crying or letting her sad thoughts overtake her. She just wanted to be a mommy so badly she could nearly taste it and yet it felt so very far away and completely out of reach. Sometimes she felt like there was this giant hole right in the center of her body, but it didn't just feel like something was missing, it felt like it ached to the point of hurting because it needed to be filled. At times when that feeling was very strong, it physically hurt and was very uncomfortable to even breathe around. It truly felt like her insides were hollowed out all the way through and knowing that it may never be filled in or the pain may never stop was very frightening.

She tried to think about something else, but it was difficult when this whole day was to celebrate mothers. Something she had desired to be since she was a little girl. It felt like a slap in the face to be thinking and hurting from the realization that she wasn't a mother daily and then to have to sit and listen to all of this for a couple of hours and realize all day that she still wasn't one. In a way, she wondered if even the daughters and mothers who were sharing their touching stories really realized what they had fully. Sure, they were grateful for each other and loved each other, but did they really know how blessed they were to have that when some women never got to experience it?

Suddenly the empty feeling along with the pain in her heart was hurting so much that Jadie could take no more. She was so grateful for her mother and while the service truly was lovely, it was just too much for her due to her current situation. She tried to appear calm and not in a rush as she left the sanctuary and headed to an empty classroom. *I hurt so badly for this each and every day and I can't just sit there and listen to that right now.* It felt like it was only making the hole inside of her even bigger and hurt even more. *Please fill it God. I realize it may not be now, but please let it be soon.*

Jadie wanted to talk to Chase after church, but she also realized there was someone else who would understand her heart who she desperately needed to talk to. Yes, a call to Amy would definitely be on the agenda for later this afternoon.

While Jadie not so patiently waited for the church service to end, she reflected back to the lovely dinner Chase had taken her out to for her birthday last month. They were simple people and didn't usually do anything extravagant, but Chase had said he'd wanted to do something special and took her to a lovely restaurant where they had to dress up quite a bit. Jadie had felt very special and loved and Chase could barely drag his eyes off of her all night for as lovely as she looked in a black evening gown and with soft curls in her hair. Their table was overlooking a bay and the lighting was soft and the music which played softly in the background was a dramatic but peaceful classical. Jadie had nearly been breathless with what a beautiful effect this all caused and had a wonderful time. The fact that their food was delicious made it an even more perfect evening. As she shared the wonderful time with her husband, her heart had hurt deeply for some of the women on her group who had shared that their husbands didn't seem to care as much about their infertility as they did. So they often felt even more alone and isolated and some couples were even getting divorced over their differences. It made Jadie appreciative of just one more thing about her husband and it made her love him all the more. She loved that he wanted a family just as much as she did and that it meant so much to him. His support also meant the world to her and she talked to him more than to any one else about their struggles and she was infinitely grateful they had that with each other.

Muffled voices and activity drifted to where Jadie was and she realized church was out. She stood and was ready to go find her husband. She couldn't wait to talk to him, and later to Amy, about how she'd been feeling. For one of the first times that day, she smiled. She was so glad she had Chase for a husband.

❤ ❤ ❤

The glass of water and light yellow, oval shaped pill sat on the bathroom sink just waiting for Jadie to take it. She had never had trouble swallowing pills before, but it was so thick in the middle that she sometimes had trouble getting it down. It often felt like it got hung up in her throat for a moment before she could get it swallowed completely and she didn't like that feeling. It felt so amazing to finally be doing something that may actually result in a baby for her and Chase. She put the pill in her mouth and tried to not psych herself out before attempting to swallow it. She was glad when it went down on the first attempt.

She had been taking them for a few days now. She started taking them the day after she ovulated just like her Doctor had instructed. The OPK's she used told her the day before she ovulated and she had gotten her positive on cycle day seventeen meaning she ovulated on cycle day eighteen. So on day nineteen she had begun taking them.

She still was amazed that such a simple solution existed for what she had. At least, what they knew was wrong so far. She was hoping and praying that this was all that was wrong and simply taking this little pill would finally give them the miracle they both so desperately wanted.

Jadie usually got tired and a bit dizzy after taking it, so she decided to read some e-mails on the computer and then do devotions. She had to be to work at noon, so she also wanted to get a couple of things done around the house before she left. She felt it was wise to do the things she could while seated first though due to the effects of the prometrium.

Jadie prayed every day that their journey would soon be over. She didn't know how people like Jake and Amy did it. There were some women on her group who had been trying for five, seven, or even ten or more years. Some couples struggled with secondary infertility, where they had previously had a child but then had trouble conceiving after that. Jadie felt so badly for them and admired them so much at the same time.

While she was online, she decided to enter some things on her chart from the past couple of days. She had avoided charting for a long time because it had seemed so overwhelming and also something she just didn't feel ready to do. But once she had started, she was amazed how quickly she picked up on it all. Now it only took her a few minutes to enter things in and she could tell just by glancing what everything meant and stood for, where she was in her cycle, and so on. The only thing she did differently now that she was on the prometrium was to enter that she was taking her meds that day. The chart added a line to the bottom that said "meds" and there was a box for each day on that line so it showed exactly when she started taking it, what days she was on it, and when she stopped. She actually enjoyed charting now. It was nice to have a place that organized everything she needed to keep track of along with her symptoms and her meds all in one convenient place. It was also neat to see her temps reflect when she ovulated along with the OPK's.

After getting done what she wanted to online, she glanced at the verses that she had printed and had taped around the computer area. She also had a piece of paper in her locker at work. It was a good reminder for her and it encouraged her daily. The most recent verse she had found just a few days ago while doing devotions that really stuck out to her was Psalm 113:9 which said, "He makes the barren woman abide in the house As a joyful mother of children. Praise the LORD!" Jadie had gotten covered in goose bumps when she read it. She and Amy had talked the next day on the phone and she asked Amy if she'd ever read it. Amy said she had and that she quoted it to herself almost daily and apologized for not telling it to Jadie sooner. Jadie didn't mind that Amy hadn't mentioned it, but it was certainly a treasure to find and words she had clung to daily since.

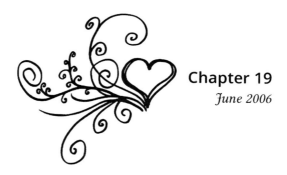

Chapter 19
June 2006

The sun beat down on Chase's bent back as he threw scrap and chunks of material from a trailer into the large dumpster at the work site. It was a fairly hot day, but Chase felt he'd grown somewhat accustomed to it since he'd been working out in the weather a lot for the past few years. He straightened for a moment and removed his work glove so he could take the cap off his bottled water to get a drink. He felt oddly energized working outside and he enjoyed his work very much. His skin seemed to eagerly soak up the sun rays as they shone down on him all day. His skin always got very dark in the summer time. He had always enjoyed summer more than Jadie. She preferred spring as she didn't care for the heat of summer.

As he cleared the remaining scrap from the trailer, Chase couldn't help but let his mind wander to the past Sunday's church service. It was Father's Day and it was much harder than he'd expected. Becoming a father was something he just always figured he'd be one day. When he'd met Jadie, he thought much more seriously about it. When they got married, it was an amazing dream and one of the things he looked most forward to about their future. Now it felt like it was a hundred miles away and he had no way to get to it. He would walk towards it and try to make progress, but he could never tell if he was getting any closer. He sighed loudly. He hated the feeling of not knowing if it would ever happen. He had never wanted something so badly in his entire life. So as he sat there and listened to people talk about it, he could only imagine it from one perspective and not the other. He did have a father, but he wasn't sure he would ever be one. Most of the time he didn't view things in a very bleak light, but he was feeling that way ever since that service. Most of the time he could convince himself, and he tried to convince Jadie, that it would happen for them . . . at least one way or another. But lately, he felt extra discouraged. He was glad they'd been to the doctor and had at least one answer, but the hope he'd felt swell from that initially had crashed like a wave that didn't have the wind to push another behind it. The first month of Jadie being on the medication hadn't worked and he was surprised at the level of hopelessness that had caused him. He tried to stay strong for Jadie, but he'd never felt more discouraged. Suddenly it had overtaken him and he felt more down about everything than he had thus far.

As he had sat through that service, the pain got so strong he wasn't sure he could bear it. He had glanced around the sanctuary and watched as proud Daddies all over were holding their babies and little ones and had a look that was a mix of love and pride that was so strong that you could see and sense it. The sight of it felt like a knife through Chase's heart. He just never thought he would be here. Through Jadie's research they had realized it was so much more common than he had once realized.

Sometimes he wished he had someone to talk to like Jadie had Amy. But he didn't know any other guys who were going through this who would understand. He had shared it with his closest friend and while he was sympathetic and Chase knew he prayed for him, he didn't have much to say about it. Chase understood, but it was hard sometimes to not have any one who had been there or was going through it to talk to.

His mind went back to the service. They had also showed a video that had brought tears to Chase's eyes. Just when he thought he could take no more, they closed the service by singing a song called "While I'm Waiting" by John Waller. It renewed his spirit some and was something he was trying very hard to commit to do in his heart. He heard the song in his head while he finished up his work:

"I'm waiting
 I'm waiting on You, Lord
 And I am hopeful
 I'm waiting on You, Lord
 Though it is painful
 But patiently, I will wait
 I will move ahead, bold and confident
 Taking every step in obedience
 While I'm waiting
 I will serve You
 While I'm waiting
 I will worship
 While I'm waiting
 I will not faint
 I'll be running the race
 Even while I wait
 I'm waiting
 I'm waiting on You, Lord
 And I am peaceful
 I'm waiting on You, Lord
 Though it's not easy
 But faithfully, I will wait
 Yes, I will wait
 I will serve You while I'm waiting
 I will worship while I'm waiting
 I will serve You while I'm waiting
 I will worship while I'm waiting
 I will serve you while I'm waiting
 I will worship while I'm waiting on You, Lord"

He closed his eyes for a moment. *Lord, I'm trying to wait on You and serve You as I should, but I'm doubting and hurting. Please help me. And please help us to have a baby soon.*

Many miles away, Jake sat at his kitchen table trying to study. He was getting so close to being a licensed electrician and he couldn't wait to have it behind him. Once he finished his classes he had an exam to take. He was attempting to get some work and studying done on both tonight while Amy was away at her women's Bible Study. But he had a hard time focusing lately and felt distracted. He shut one of his books with a sigh and then rested his head in his hands.

He and Amy had continued to talk and mourn over their decision to not pursue more treatments to have biological children. While they both knew it was the right thing, it was still a difficult time. Mother's Day had been particularly hard on Amy and if he was honest, this Father's Day had been one of the roughest days he had had as well. He and Amy had found another couple at their church who was also going through infertility and they had spoken with them after the Father's Day service. They were all saying how services like that made them feel extremely isolated and very different from everyone else who attended and how that could be rough. Jake felt like a minority amongst everyone else and it was rough for him. It made him feel like he wasn't as much of a man or like something was wrong with him. While deep down he knew that wasn't true and he tried to not dwell on it, there were times he felt that way.

It had been a long road and one that consumed both he and Amy much of the time. He was a hundred times more ready to have this part of his life behind him than he was the years of work and study towards becoming an electrician. He hoped that their journey was nearly over and that they would have children of their own soon. They were nearly finished with the myriad of paperwork, home studies, and other things that went along with becoming foster parents. Since that seemed to be the cheapest and most efficient way to get to adoption, he was hoping that they would be on their way towards that soon. He was becoming more and more at peace all the time with adopting instead of having biological children. He had always thought adoption would be something he and Amy would strongly consider, but he always assumed they would have at least one or two of their own children as well. He was getting used to the idea that adoption was their only way to have children now.

He wanted to be a father so badly that he knew that whether Amy had carried the child or not didn't matter to him. He would love them with his whole heart. He only hoped he had that opportunity soon. Very soon.

He got up and got a glass of water and prayed to give himself a moment to regroup. Then he sat back down at the table with purpose. He had an hour until Amy got home and he wanted to get a lot done in that time. With new resolve he opened his book again and set to work.

♥ ♥ ♥

Kendra looked down at her ever expanding middle. She gently caressed her tummy and felt her baby gently kick in response. She couldn't stop her grin. She was twenty-two weeks pregnant now and still in awe that she and Daniel finally had their miracle baby on the way. They'd decided to not find out the gender and be surprised at the birth. But they did have a nurse write the gender of the baby on a card and it was in an envelope and under their mattress at home in case they changed their minds. Kendra knew she could hold out, but she wasn't so sure about Daniel. She had never seen him so excited and it touched her beyond words. She would never forget the look on his face when she'd told him. It had broken her heart over the years every time she'd had to tell him that that month too was a failure. He'd even cried a couple of times when she'd told him and to see those tears running down her strong soldier's face, who wanted nothing more than to be a daddy, had absolutely broken her heart. So to finally be able to give him the amazing news was so sweet and rewarding. It was one of the happiest moments of her life. While pregnancy did have some not so pleasant aspects, Kendra never complained. She had waited years for this opportunity and one she wasn't sure she'd ever have. So to get to experience it herself was incredible. She and Daniel had decided to try IVF twice and if it didn't work then they would have moved on to surrogacy and tried as many times as it took. So while she was not overly worried about never having a child of her own, she was sad at the thought that she may never get to experience pregnancy or birth. She thanked God daily for the miracle of life and the very special role she got to play in that.

Emma watched Kendra gently caress her sweet little baby bump and then smile. She was genuinely happy for her friend. They had continued to grow closer over the months and even e-mailed and occasionally talked on the phone outside of work. But Emma couldn't help but get choked up. She knew now she would never experience what Kendra was right now and it nearly killed her every time she thought about it. She and Steve had lost their seventh baby at about four weeks last month and had seriously prayed and talked since. Just last week they had decided that they would no longer try to have children of their own. They had spoken with their doctor and despite having tried different medicines to help, nothing had worked. Other than a slightly odd shaped uterus, they couldn't nail down why Emma was unable to carry babies. They didn't feel her uterus would be a problem until later in the pregnancy, but they felt confident she would get far enough along that the baby would not need to stay in the NICU. But they were either wrong or something else was going on that was preventing it from happening. The Doctor had encouraged them to consider adoption or some other option as they said it would get harder on Emma's body to continue to take recurring miscarriages. The night they had decided Emma had cried until she was sick to her stomach and then cried some more. Steve just held her and let tears of his own slide down his cheeks as their hearts broke in unison. She couldn't imagine never having a child of her own. The pain was just too much to bear. She had been since working to come to grips with it, but it was still an extremely emotional and difficult time. To her it felt worse than someone she loved dying. She was mourning children she would never get to meet, know, or raise. She was mourning her dreams of being a mother. Her heart was still way too raw to even begin to think about adoption or some other option.

She quickly wiped at the tears that had spilled over and were running down her face, but still opened her top desk drawer. In it she had a frame for each of her seven babies that she lost. She knew most people would think she was crazy, but she had known which gender each of her babies were. She and Steve had also both had dreams about them and in a few of the dreams the babies' names were revealed. The other ones they named as well. She had hand painted each frame in bright colors and had stenciled each baby's name across the tops of the frames. Most of the frames held a picture of her positive pregnancy test with that baby. One held a picture the Doctor had taken measuring the heartbeat. The baby just looked like a small blob on the screen and then the bottom had the wavelengths of the heartbeat. And for two of them she had an ultrasound picture, so that is what the frame held for those babies. They'd had four boys and three little girls. Each with their own names and she would never forget them. For now she kept the frames at work, but eventually she would move them back home and place them around their bedroom. For now she didn't want to think about any one seeing them and questioning her or Steve about it.

Emma wasn't sure she could ever explain the pain of a miscarriage to anyone. The love she had for those babies was so great she couldn't put it into words. What was for many people the happiest times of their lives, Emma and Steve always had ripped away from them. They never got to know their baby, see them for the first time, hold them, or take them home from the hospital. Emma never even got to experience pregnancy very far which she would have loved to do. What would she have looked like with a "baby bump" as many women affectionately called their ever-growing middles? What would it have felt like to feel her baby move inside of her? But even though she and Steve hadn't experienced those things, the love that a parent felt for a child was still there and then so was the mourning when that child was gone. It would be hard to describe to someone how you could have that amazing joy at having a child and the intense love for the sweet little one that came with it, only to have it taken away from you. The pain was so intense that Emma could feel it physically just thinking about it. Her heart felt broken and she felt certain in that moment, as she caressed each of her sweet babies' pictures with tear-filled eyes, that no one could ever understand entirely unless they had been there themselves. Walking by baby sections at stores was something that most people who were pregnant or were looking forward to having children got excited by. For people like Emma, it was another heartbreaking reminder of all she could have had with her babies, but never got to experience. Emma once again wiped at her tears and gently slid the drawer shut.

Later that day Kendra and Emma talked on one of their breaks. Kendra was always very sensitive and never mentioned her pregnancy or the baby unless Emma brought it up. Emma was genuinely excited for Kendra, but there were particularly painful moments where she didn't care to talk about it. She appreciated how much Kendra understood more than she could ever say. This was one of the days that Emma didn't ask. After looking at all she had to cherish of her little ones she'd lost she couldn't bear to talk about a thriving pregnancy without bursting into tears. Instead she decided to share the good news she and Steve had decided on not long after their other big decision.

"Well, I have something big to share."

Kendra's eyes sparkled. "What is it? Don't leave me in

suspense!"

Emma laughed. "Steve and I have been feeling led in this direction for awhile now and in light of our decision we feel the timing is right. We've been praying about it and we've decided to pursue becoming missionaries."

Kendra's eyes grew large and then she smiled and hugged her friend. "I'm really happy for you guys! I'm just bummed because if you go somewhere far away I'm going to miss you!"

Emma was still taken aback at times by Kendra's openness, but she cherished it all the same. "I will miss you too! We already called a highly recommended missionary agency last night and they are already looking things over and we have a meeting scheduled for next week."

"Wow! Well, how exciting! If this is what God wants you to do, I know He'll bless it."

Emma smiled. "Thank you, Kendra. That means a lot to me."

Emma was still getting used to the idea and everything seemed to be moving quickly. But Kendra was right. God would bless them and be with them, so she had nothing to fear.

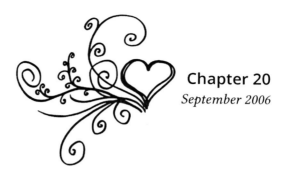

Chapter 20
September 2006

Amy could hardly believe that it'd been three days ago that she'd gotten the call. She had been dusting and trying to get her cleaning done since it was her day off at the library when the phone had rang. She'd barely gotten to it before the person hung up. It was their adoption case worker, Doreen, and after saying hello, she dove right into the news she had. "Alright, Amy, here's the deal. We have two little girls for you if you're interested. They're roughly six months old and a year-and-a-half old. Their names are Meg and Maddie. They have been taken out of their mother's custody and we need to place them with someone immediately. If you're interested, we would be bringing them to you on Monday."

During the quick, but information-filled few sentences, Amy had literally dropped her duster, was standing stock still with her eyes open wide, and couldn't think of a thing to say. *Two little girls? Two precious little girls? Monday? Were they interested?* Her heart beat so hard and she knew immediately they were interested; it just felt so surreal and out of the blue! She knew when they got a placement it would be similar to this; she and Jake just weren't expecting to get a placement so soon.

"Amy, are you there?"

"Umm . . . yes! Sorry . . . I am just shocked. I . . . uh . . . need to talk to Jake. How soon do you need an answer by?"

"By the end of the day. If you are unable to take them, we need to work on finding someone else."

"Okay, I will call Jake right now and let you know as soon as possible."

"Okay, Amy, I will talk to you later today then."

"Yes. Umm . . . thank you."

The phone call ended as abruptly as it had begun and Amy still had felt completely in shock. She and Jake had talked, prayed, and decided within a matter of minutes to say yes. So Amy had called Doreen back right away and let her know they wanted to take them.

The next few days passed in a flurry of activity as she and Jake got ready for the girls. They had made a couple of shopping trips to get more items they needed since they knew the girls' ages (they had accumulated some things just to be prepared since getting licensed as foster parents) as well as lots of phone calls to family, more last minute planning and preparations, and so on. Amy had of course called Jadie that Friday evening and her friend was ecstatic! Amy and Jake were thrilled too, but it also was still sinking in and felt a bit surreal. Amy couldn't help but wonder how her heart would take it if the girls were taken away from them after a time. But she and Jake had talked and prayed a lot about it and they knew God was in control.

During all of the preparations for the girls, Jake had also completed his last requirements and received his electrician's license. Amy was immensely proud and they managed to have a family dinner with all of Jake's side of the family to celebrate. Jake and Amy both were so relieved to have the stress and extra work he had been through behind them. The timing also was amazing because now that that was completed and behind them, they could focus on the girls.

After one last inspection by Amy to make sure the girls' room was completely prepared for their arrival, they were now on their way to meet up with Doreen and get the girls. It was early evening and they were meeting her at a park. Typically she would have brought the girls right to their home, but she had another placement to do yet that evening, so this would save her time. Amy and Jake had done a lot of careful research and chosen just the right car seats which were all installed and ready to go in their backseat. She and Jake held hands, but didn't talk overly much. She knew they were both equal parts excited and nervous. In a way they were about to become parents in an instant even though they didn't know if these little girls would be staying with them permanently or not.

When they got to the park, Amy noticed her hands were trembling, but she couldn't help but smile. She had prayed for years to have children in her home and to be a mother, and in a way, her prayers would be answered in a few minutes. She tried to not get her hopes up, but she wanted these little girls to be her daughters and to know they were her's forever. She tried to check herself and prayed inwardly that God's will would be done and that no matter what happened, she and Jake would take good care of the little girls and show them God's love in whatever amount of time they had them.

She and Jake shared a knowing smile and joined hands as they walked towards a group of picnic tables where Doreen was sitting. She had the older little girl in her lap and was holding the baby in her other arm. A bag or two sat next to her on the bench which Amy presumed was the few things they had been using to care for the girls over the past few days and a few personal possessions. The closer they got, the more Amy felt her heart respond to the beautiful little girls. The older one seemed so tiny to Amy and had blonde hair and delicate features. She peered over the blanket that covered part of the baby's face and saw that she had similar features to her sister but had light brown hair. They both were fair skinned and beautiful. They also seemed very vulnerable to Amy in that moment which made her "mother hen" tendencies kick in and helped some of her own feelings of vulnerability dissipate. She and Jake both smiled sweetly at the girls and said hello. The older of the two ducked her head shyly and sucked harder on her pacifier which she had just placed in her mouth.

Amy couldn't believe the amount of love and protectiveness she felt instantly for the little girls and from stealing a glance at her husband, it was clear by the look on his face and especially the light in his eyes that he felt the same way. After talking to Doreen for fifteen or twenty minutes and getting more details about them, Amy and Jake each took one of the little girls and carried them to their car to go home. She was sure it was awkward for the older girl, Meg, to be carried by a stranger, but she didn't cry. The brave little sweetheart! Amy couldn't wait to wipe away the look of fear and uncertainty from the little girls' precious faces in the next few days.

Amy once again was overcome by how surreal it was and how much her heart wanted to take off without her as she looked in the rearview mirror at the two special little girls. Especially when little Meg reached over and took her sister's little hand in her own. Amy's eyes filled with tears and she gave Jake's hand a squeeze. She suddenly had no doubts that she could care for these little girls. She had babysat younger children as a teen and had helped her sister plenty of times with her nieces. She just wanted to erase whatever hurts their little hearts had suffered and love them the way that no one ever had. The desire to have these girls remain in their lives and hearts forever increased practically by the second. Again Amy prayed that God would help her to survive if it wasn't His plan for them to stay with them. But already Amy prayed that it would be. She and Jake talked for a few minutes about their feelings, prayed aloud, and then Amy glanced again in the rearview mirror at the now two sleeping angels in her backseat. Her heart swelled and she prayed that she wasn't looking at just any little girls. She prayed she was looking at her daughters.

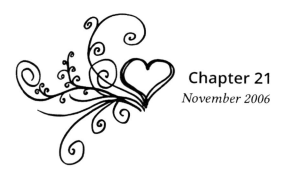

Chapter 21
November 2006

The foggy mist filled a small circle on the window and then mostly dissipated as Jadie drew long breaths in and out while staring out her bedroom window. Outside everything seemed so dead and lifeless and in some ways Jadie felt like it reflected her mood. Their infertility was especially hard on Chase lately and it was so hard to see her normally happy and confident husband struggling so much. His pain almost seemed greater than her's at this point as God had given her a peace that truly did pass understanding. It still hurt and it was still hard for her, but somehow He had given her the strength to go on and a peace and even joy to sustain her through daily life. She was so grateful for it and was amazed that right when she felt like she couldn't go on or take another step, God had gifted her with the grace to make it through.

But now her heart was heavy for her husband and for the burden they both still faced. No matter how much she tried not to, Jadie dreaded with every fiber of her being the tests that seemed to loom ahead of them if they didn't get pregnant on their own. This was their last month of medicine and then it was back to the specialist to proceed with testing. It was the most intense and pressure-filled two week wait she had experienced thus far. Without the peace God had given her, she would have been ripping her hair out with the insane amount of stress of it all. The peace made it tolerable and she prayed daily for that same thing for her hurting husband.

Her chin was rested on her crossed arms as she sat on her knees on the floor and continued to look out the window. Would the sound of children's laughter drifting in the windows ever be heard? Would her children ever climb the tree that grew taller each year or carve their initials into it's tough bark with a knife? Or would everything outside just always look empty and hollow like it did now? Would that tree ever bear the marks that she hoped it would or have a swing hanging from it? Would she see it and have memories of her children climbing it? Or would it always be as it was now: bare and leafless, it's empty branches reaching into the sky? It seemed to represent infertility so well as it stood alone, empty, and stretching into the cloudy sky. She continued to stare and wonder. Would she and Chase sit on either side of their house watching their children play in the front or back yard someday or would they be rocking, old and gray, and staring at the same emptiness with it reflecting heavily in their hearts? No children or grandchildren to visit, to call, or to share holidays or memories with. Just them rocking for years on end as the seasons and years passed by. Just barrenness, like the tree. Not that Chase wasn't enough for her, but she wanted to have a family with him so badly she physically ached. Jadie's eyes filled with tears and she forced herself to move away from the window.

Two years was such a long time. The second had been harder than the first. So many months of waiting, wondering, and pain. Having children was such a natural and simple part of life for most people. If a couple wanted children, they had a family. So why were she and Chase so backwards? Familiar negative thoughts assaulted her like *"would we not make good parents?"* and *"are we being punished for something?"* She felt the weight of discouragement on her like a heavy burden and it felt as though she couldn't move. She could not allow herself to think that way. She reminded herself of Jeremiah 29:11—a verse she and Chase clung to lately. "'For I know the plans I have for you,' declares the LORD, 'plans for welfare and not for calamity to give you a future and a hope'." She quickly went to their bed and dropped to her knees; her burden too heavy to carry alone. She folded her hands and prayed: "Dear Heavenly Father, help me to remember those words: a future and hope. I know You have amazing plans for us even though it's so hard for Chase and I right now to know what those are or to remain positive about whatever they may be. But You are wise and all-knowing and I know You love us with a love we cannot even begin to comprehend. You are not doing this to hurt us and You do love us. Two years have gone by, Lord, since we've been trying to make a baby. It's so hard to wonder day in and day out if it's ever going to happen for us. It hurts so badly. I've never experienced such pain. But I know You understand and You care. I just ask now, Lord, that you would fill my heart with the peace You've been giving me recently. Help me God to make it through this. I can't do it alone! Please encourage and comfort Chase's heart as well right now, Lord. He's having such a hard time. I know only You can give Him that indescribable peace. And Lord, please give us a baby, I beg of You. Maybe it's wrong to ask that way, but I feel free to come to You with my heart's deepest desire and ask for it now. I know You will give it in your timing if You choose to. Please let that peace continue to wash over me. I love you. In Jesus' Name, Amen." Immediately when she opened her eyes, she felt the burden lift and peace circulate in her chest and around her heart. She felt lighter and full of a joy that she knew came from above. The amazing feeling made her eyes grow teary and she was so thankful for God's tender mercies towards her. She and Chase would be a family just the two of them or adopt if they never had biological children. It would hurt to never have biological children, but there were still possibilities for them. After reflecting for a few more minutes, she decided to call Amy. A chat with her dearest friend would do her a lot of good.

Her friend answered on the second ring and Jadie smiled,

the way she always did when she heard her voice.

"Hey! Not a bad time is it?"

Jadie could hear the smile in her friend's voice as she responded, "Of course not! Never for you!"

Jadie shared some about her sad thoughts earlier and how she'd prayed and now felt better.

"God is so good to us. I am just sorry Chase is still having a hard time. People think infertility isn't as hard on men, but it really is! I will pray for him."

"Thanks, Amy. And I agree it is just as hard on them."

"So you said you're in your two week wait and then it is back to the Doctor, but I can't remember, how many months have you been on the prometrium now?"

"Six. She prescribed enough for four months, but there were extra pills in each 'month' if that makes sense."

"Yes, it does. So are you still having lots of false symptoms?"

Jadie couldn't help but sigh. "Yes, and it has been so hard at times. Some months it feels like I have a million pregnancy symptoms and then I just want to go crazy when the test comes up negative just like it always does. The last cycle I was on it my stomach even swelled and I couldn't help but hold my hands over it and wonder what it would be like if there was really a baby in there."

Amy's heart broke over her friend's admission and her tone. "Oh honey, I'm sorry! I know that's so awful to be given false hope and have it taken away. I know at times this has been so torturous for you."

"Thanks. I just thought this was going to be an easy fix, but here we are six months later and still not pregnant. On top of it, the false symptoms have just about made me go crazy at times! You know how badly I do not want to do any testing, but at the same time I am relieved that this is my last month on it for now. I probably sound so ungrateful! I wanted a treatment and now that I'm doing it I'm complaining about it. I don't mean to, it's just been hard."

"You don't sound ungrateful at all! Treatment is not easy. Especially not when it involves hormones and messes with our already sensitive emotions over such a sensitive issue as trying to have a baby. It's a big deal! And it's okay to not be rejoicing in how hard getting treated can be."

"I'm glad you understand. And I am grateful, honestly! I just was hoping this was going to be all that was wrong and we would just treat it and finally get pregnant. After six months, it's not really looking that way." She sighed. "We'll see."

Amy sighed as well. "I know. I was hoping this was going to be it for you too. And I still am! There's still hope. You never know! Jake and I are praying."

"Thanks. Yeah, I know there is. It's just a hard line to find between not getting your hopes up and still having hope."

Amy couldn't resist laughing and Jadie knew she wasn't laughing at her. "I know just what you mean!"

Jadie smiled too. "Even though it's still hard, this peace God has been giving me just helps so much! I can't imagine being where we are right now in our journey without it. I was just thinking earlier I'd be ripping my hair out!"

"Yes, God is good to get us through the hard times. And I know just what you mean! There have been times that if He didn't carry me through I'm sure I would have been completely bald."

They shared a laugh.

"I am still just so proud of Jake for getting his electrician's license. He worked so hard! Is he glad it's behind him?"

"Me too and yes, he's very glad!"

"And do you have any updates for me on the girls' case? I haven't talked to you since our e-mail the other day."

"Hmm . . . well, we have a court date coming up in just a couple of days. I'm not sure what all it will entail. I'll make sure to update you when we get home."

"Okay, you do that! And I'll be praying in the meantime."

"Thanks!"

"No problem. So I still can't get over the fact that Emma from the group will be heading off for the mission field soon! She seems so excited."

Amy agreed. "And I am still blown away that her and Kendra worked together all that time and didn't realize they knew each other from the group! I just think it's so great how they are good friends now. You can tell from their responses to each other on the group."

"Yeah, kind of like us! It's amazing the bonds you can form with people you've never met 'in real life'. That was just such a God thing how they knew each other that whole time!"

"Oh yeah, it definitely was! And you're right. I always felt connected to the women on the group because of what we had in common, but I had never developed a close friendship with someone from the Internet until you. It's amazing really!"

"It is, and I'm so glad I found you!"

Amy's heart was warmed by her friend's sweet words and tone. "Me too! You have no idea how much!"

They talked more about a few girls from the group who were having a particularly hard time and Jadie asked about Maddie and Meg. They finished up by again promising to pray for each other and promising to update one another as soon as they knew something.

Jadie felt happy after hanging up. She always did after talking to Amy. She prayed right then and thanked God for giving her such an amazing friend. She also prayed for Chase again as she knew he would be sad when he came home from work, like he had been lately. She also knew they may end up talking more about how this month marked two years for them. It still felt surreal in a way, but the pain reminded her it was true and it was really happening to them. But God would get them through and she determined to remind her husband of that and of how they would get through this together.

♥ ♥ ♥

The courtroom didn't have a lot of people in it, but it still felt like a small space to Amy. It felt uncomfortable to her to be around the woman who was the biological mother of the girls Amy already considered to be her's in a way. Amy and Jake had decided to follow all the court proceedings for the mother of the girls even though they weren't required to. They wanted to be aware of all that was going on and the way to stay best informed was to come themselves. At the same time, Amy knew that the mother had to have figured out who they were by now and that made Amy feel self-conscious. She knew now that the woman's name was Linda. She seemed too thin to Amy and was a few years younger than her. She had long brown hair which was pulled back in a pony tail and she was somewhat tall and thin. She seemed strangely disconnected from everything and very serious, but Amy could see the pain deep in her eyes. In a way she felt sorry for Linda. She wondered what had happened in her life to make her not try harder to take care of her children. Amy had no desire to judge the woman and in fact had been praying for her since the day the girls had gotten placed with them.

It was such a mess to try to sort out in her mind. On the one hand Amy couldn't wait for her rights to be terminated and the girls to officially become part of her and Jake's family. On the other hand, she did feel sorry for Linda and wished that she was raising her own children and that they could be with their mother. Amy also felt frustrated that the courts had already given Linda so many chances when she continued to fail to provide for her children, but on the other hand did believe in forgiveness, second chances, and people changing. But how many chances should someone have? Especially when children's lives and well-being were in the balance. It was not an easy decision to be sure. Since it was such a serious issue, she guessed that was why a biological parent was given so many chances. But to Amy who loved the girls furiously already, part of her was angry that they were allowed to stay in a bad situation. She knew there were no easy answers to problems like these, but she hoped that what was best for the girls would be done now. Amy was already too in love for her heart to allow her to wish for anything other than the girls to become a permanent part of she and Jake's family. She also strongly believed that was what was best for the girls. Another thing that Amy tried to wrap her mind around was how someone could time and time again do the same things knowing that they could lose their own children. Amy wanted children so badly and couldn't imagine doing that. She again tried to not judge Linda; it was just something she didn't really understand. It also made Amy feel guilty knowing that she was wishing children away from their biological mother when she would have given anything to have children of her own. It just felt strange to her and something she had a hard time settling her feelings about. But it was important that the girls have a good life and Amy always wanted to remember to remain compassionate to Linda and pray for her no matter what happened.

Amy and Jake's concern right now was that Linda's rights may not get terminated. Even if that happened there was always a chance that a family member could step forward and want the children placed with them. The biological father was not an issue as he had apparently willingly signed his rights away awhile ago and from what Samantha (one of the people they dealt with through the adoption agency) told them, he had no interest in trying to get his rights back. She and Jake were just praying for the Lord's will, which they were hoping was that the girls be placed with them.

Amy tried to follow everything the best she could. It was strange to her how many times the court would be meeting with the mother before moving ahead on things. She had learned so much since she and Jake had started doing foster care. Things had been immensely complicated and involved and she had learned a lot about a lot of things. She also had learned that everything took a long time to process and go through the proper channels. They had been told that pursuing foster care was the best and cheapest way to get to adoption and their adoption worker had told them that was usually the case. She and Jake could have chosen to only get children placed with them whose parental rights had already been terminated, but they had prayed about it and felt led to accept either. They also had been more lenient on what age they preferred than Amy had originally felt they would. But by doing those two things, they had increased their odds of getting placements faster. Now that they had the girls, she knew they had done the right thing and the Lord had His hand on it all.

Once court was adjourned, Amy was relieved to get outside in the fresh air. It was chilly, but still nice to be out especially since the sun was shining. She and Jake talked to their case worker for a few minutes and made sure they had written down the next date Linda would need to be in court and then headed to their car hand-in-hand. Amy wondered how long this road would be for them, but tried not to fret. She knew that the Lord knew what He was doing and she just had to keep trusting. Her time through infertility had shown her that He was always right there, even if things didn't work out the way she felt they should. He loved them and had better plans for them than they had for themselves. It didn't mean things weren't hard sometimes or that she didn't worry, but she worked on keeping her focus on the Lord. He would see them through.

Chapter 22

Emma sat at her small kitchen table drumming her fingers on the hard surface. Steve would be getting home from work in about an hour and she'd already started dinner, so for now she just sat alone with her thoughts. There were times when she'd lost her babies that she felt the pain would suffocate her or take her over and there would be nothing of her left. Her heart was still healing, but she was amazed how much some time had done. She still wished it hadn't happened and she still thought about all seven of her babies and missed them daily. But God had begun to restore her and it was such a relief to no longer be bogged down by such intense grief. But something Emma had pushed to the back of her mind was where her babies were now. She always thought of them at peace, but she always blocked the picture of them being in heaven from her mind. She had only thought about it a few times early on, but the last time was bombarded by intense feelings towards God. Like how could He take them for Himself when He already had plenty of people in heaven? These were Emma's only children after all and was God so selfish that He needed them with Him instead of allowing them to be with her? She had been frightened to realize how angry she was and for thinking of God, who had given His own perfect Son's life in exchange for hers and many others, as selfish. So she had put up a mental block so to speak and never allowed those thoughts in her mind again. She wouldn't allow something to come between her and her loving God and she couldn't take a chance that thinking on that would stir up those feelings again. So she hadn't thought about it since she lost her second child. Until today.

She and Kendra had been talking after work after the other employees had gone home for the day. She was feeling emotional and while crying was telling Kendra how much it hurt to know she'd never have children of her own. Kendra had let a few of her own tears slip and held Emma while she had cried. But when Kendra pulled back she looked a little sad, but mostly peaceful and a bit surprised. Emma didn't have time to question her friend about it before Kendra nearly immediately told her what she was thinking. Her voice was sincere and although she spoke softly, she nearly held an urgent tone. "But don't you see Emma? You do have children. God created seven beautiful little miracles. And while you aren't getting to raise them here on Earth, God did not create them for nothing. They are just in heaven waiting for you and Steve to one day join them. God didn't take them from you to be cruel; He just wanted heaven to be extra special for you so He has seven children waiting for you. I bet He smiles every day thinking about how happy you'll be when you meet them all one day." A couple of tears slid down her cheeks as Kendra shared her heart with her friend.

The truth of what her friend had said sent chills up and down Emma's arms and as soon as Kendra had finished speaking, Emma collapsed into her arms and sobbed softly. When she could catch her breath she told Kendra that was the most beautiful thing she'd ever heard and thanked her from the bottom of her heart for sharing that with her. Emma felt suddenly lighter and more at peace than she'd been in a long time. It suddenly dawned on her that not only did she have seven precious children in heaven, but that her children would never have to cry or be sick or feel pain. God and Jesus were their parents and there were myriads of other perfect people loving them in a way that Emma could only imagine right now. Suddenly she felt very selfish for wishing them to this sinful Earth when God had been so wonderful to not only bless her with seven sweet children, but give them a perfect life with Him right from the beginning. All this time in the back of her mind she'd thought of her lost babies as a gift not only lost, but taken. Now she realized with blinding clarity that they were gifts that were gained and that she would receive when she reached heaven one day. She was so touched she had to remind herself to breathe normally. She couldn't wait to get home and tell Steve what she had come to realize. Emma felt nearly weightless and realized this was by far one of the happiest moments of her life.

After sharing all these thoughts with a teary Kendra, Emma added something else she'd just realized.

"Did you know Kendra, that in the Bible there is this special number that is used many times? Many Pastors have said it is a symbol of completion."

Kendra thought for just a moment and then it was her turn to break out in goose bumps. She smiled slightly. "It wouldn't happen to be seven would it?"

Emma could only nod and grin for all she was worth.

Kendra hugged her friend again and then searched in her purse for a Kleenex.

"Well now that we're both a mess!" Emma laughed and accepted the Kleenex Kendra offered her. Kendra continued, "I need to get home to Daniel and Blake. Blake doesn't always take a bottle so well since he prefers the real deal, so I don't want to leave Daniel stranded if he needs help." They shared a laugh and then headed to their vehicles with promises of talking later.

Emma smiled and suddenly wanted to get up and pace the room because she was so excited and could hardly wait for Steve to get home. Instead she forced herself to remain calm and got herself a glass of ice water. She had no more than taken the first sip when she jumped as the phone rang. She sat the glass down and placed a hand over her chest. "Boy, did that about scare me out of my own skin!"

She rushed over and answered it and heard an unfamiliar male voice on the other line.

"Hello, Mrs. Simmons?"

"Yes?"

"This is Adam Johnson from Go Ye Therefore Missionary Agency."

"Oh yes, hello Mr. Johnson."

"I hope you and Steve are well."

"We are, thank you. And you?"

"I am well, thanks, and am very excited to be making this call."

"Oh?"

Emma was very curious what this was about and dropped into the nearest chair.

"Yes! I have some great news for you and your husband. As you know, the meetings we've had with you both have went very well and we've been looking into some kind of placement for you. We think the perfect thing has come up. We had a couple who was on the fence if you will, about taking on an assignment we had for them. So instead of them raising money individually for themselves, they gave it to us and we placed it in an account to be used by whoever ended up taking the assignment. They were very open about not being sure about it and they were actually trying to start a family. They felt that God would answer their prayers one way or another. Either they would get pregnant and they would know the timing wasn't right for them right now or if they didn't they would go on the trip. We preferred that the couple that goes on this assignment not have children, at least for the first couple of years so that they can fully focus on the children."

Emma's pulse had picked up considerably and she was trying to take everything in. But children? What was the assignment?

Adam continued. "Well I received a call from the couple today saying that they are about eight weeks pregnant and have taken a great deal of time to pray about it and feel this is their answer and that the timing is not right for them right now. They understandably want to focus on their own family for a few years. So now the position is open and we need a couple who is ready to start in the next four months or so. Over eighty percent of the funds have already been raised for what you would need for your first term. I apologize; I am so excited and rambling here! Do you have any questions so far?"

Emma blinked rapidly and tried to clear her head. She wanted to respond that she had about three dozen questions but tried to focus.

"Umm . . . Yes, I suppose I do. So you have this opening that we can take, but what is the assignment and where? What does it entail?"

Adam laughed. "Good questions! I suppose I should have included that in my description of everything. I just got so excited about how this came about. Okay, it's an orphanage in the Philippines. It is run right now by volunteers, but they would love to have a couple there full time. The community is very involved with it and so it would not only be a ministry to the children, but a huge outreach opportunity as well. Steve's main role would be administrative duties as well as heading up mentoring, and doing Bible studies and chapels for the children. You would help with the studies and mentoring alongside him, but would mainly be working in the children's rooms all day. They have structured activities as well as schooling depending on the age groups and of course need a chaperone as well. You both would live in the same building, but there is an apartment so to speak that is off on it's own. You will be working a lot of hours both daytimes and evenings, but you will always have about four to five hours off a day and every other weekend."

The excitement in Adam's voice was contagious and Emma was so thrilled she could hardly sit still.

"It sounds . . . amazing, Mr. Johnson."

He cut in, "Please, call me Adam."

"Okay . . . Adam. But of course my husband and I will need more details and time to pray and decide."

"Of course, we'd love to have a meeting with you as soon as possible."

"Okay, that sounds fantastic! Once we've had the meeting how long will we have to decide?"

"Well, we'd like to have a firm decision no later than a month from now because if you and Steve decide not to take it, we need time to line someone else up."

Everything was happening so quickly! Emma tried to stay focused on the matter at hand. "I understand. Thank you so much for calling us and considering us for such a great opportunity."

"My pleasure! Would you like to schedule the meeting now, or do you want to consult with Steve first?"

"No, I pretty much know his schedule, so I can schedule it now. I'm positive he's going to want to get all the details before making a decision either way."

Once Emma had made the appointment and placed the phone back on the receiver, she once again sank down into the chair. She bowed her head and prayed thanking God for his faithfulness and many blessings.

Suddenly the front door opened. "Steve!" she squealed as she rushed over to him. His eyes grew wide and he smiled. "That excited to see me?"

"Of course! But it's not just that. I have so much to tell you! Please, come sit down with me."

Two hours later, dinner had been turned to simmer and long forgotten and they had discussed both of the wonderful things that Emma had to share. They had both laughed and shed a few tears of joy. Now Emma was curled up on the couch that she hadn't moved from for the past couple of hours, and was snuggled on her husband's chest with his arm around her. In a way it felt ironic to Emma that a baby being on the way for the other couple was what was changing things for them so fast. But then, children had been a prominent thing in their lives for quite some time now. She was seeing that God used waiting for children, losing children, or children who needed parents and all children in general very much in His infinite plans.

She smiled broadly. God had blessed them so much! She and Steve both were excited to someday meet their biological children, but for now it sounded like they may have many many heart children who needed them in the Philippines. Emma and Steve could hardly wait to meet them!

♥ ♥ ♥

Kendra too was snuggled up on her husband in their living room about twenty miles away. She had shared the conversation that she and Emma had after work with Daniel and now they were curled up on the couch watching TV after dinner. Blake was nearby in his bouncer and appeared to be watching the TV as well. He was content now that he'd had what he wanted from mommy as well as his evening bath. He was all snuggled in some soft, footed jammies and was happy to try to look around and take everything in. He was such a good baby and Kendra felt like she would never tire of staring at him countless times a day. He was such a miracle and she thanked God daily for giving her such an amazing blessing. One of her favorite verses that she had printed and had alongside Blake's picture in a double frame at work was Psalm 127:3: "Behold, children are a gift of the LORD, the fruit of the womb is a reward." She loved reading all the verses in the Bible about what a blessing children were. Every time she read them it was as if her soul itself resonated with agreement.

Daniel was thinking about how it was impossible to love his little family any more than he did. He kissed Kendra's forehead and sent up a silent prayer thanking God for her and Blake. When he had found the Lord, he felt fearful that Kendra may never accept Him as he had. He had always loved his wife very much, but the changes in her since she'd given her life to Christ were astounding. They enjoyed growing together in their spiritual lives, but the unexpected extra tenderness and sweetness it had brought out in his wife had been such a blessing. He was so glad they were on the right track before they'd had Blake. Sure, they would have loved him before and been good parents and taken good care of him. But now he felt they were trying to be the kind of parents God wanted them to be and their son would be raised in the light of His truth. Daniel was convinced there was no better way to live.

Kendra smiled just as Daniel released a contented sigh.

"What's the smile for?"

"What's the sigh for?"

They both laughed.

"You go first." she insisted.

"I was just thinking about how blessed I am, how I love both of you so much, and how glad I am we have the Lord in our lives now."

Kendra's smile filled her face. "Mmhhmm."

"Your turn."

"I am just so glad how the talk with Emma went today. She was just so happy and excited about it. But beyond that, I just have a feeling that God is going to do something really big using those two and has something really good planned for them, you know?"

Daniel smiled. "I'm sure. And for us too, honey. For us too."

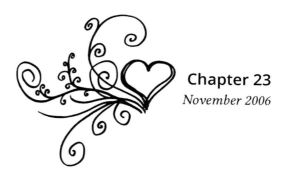

Chapter 23
November 2006

Peace and pacing were two things that consumed Jadie as she anxiously waited. She had been on the prometrium for six months now. It took her a few months to learn that she could no longer trust the signs and signals that her body gave her. She had done research on prometrium and understood why some women could not bear to be on it. It had been agonizing to have pregnancy symptoms and even have her stomach bloat and get hard as if she had a slight baby bump. Charting daily all of her symptoms on top of that nearly drove her mad at times. Having to think about it several times a day and be so consumed with it even when she didn't want to be on top of the physical symptoms she was experiencing had been very stressful at times. She and Chase had decided to take one cycle off this past month just for the sake of her sanity and to re-group. But now here they were, on their very last cycle of prometrium. So much rested on this! If this didn't work, it was time to head back to the fertility specialist for more tests and more waiting and wondering. Jadie knew she could and would do that if she had to, but there were times she just wanted to hide and not have to even think about facing that after all they'd already been through. She would be elated if she didn't have to face that. Jadie marveled at the strength of Amy and other women on her group who went through more years, more testing, more treatment, and much more waiting than she had. It could all be so much to bear. Jadie wondered often how any one did it without God in their life. There were times that she felt if she hadn't had Him to lean on that she would have come undone at the seams and completely unraveled.

Two years had passed since she and Chase had sat on their bed dreaming and praying about starting their family. Life had gone on, but in that one respect they seemed frozen in time. She sometimes felt like the animals that had gotten frozen in ice. She was stock still, but everything still went on around her. Her infertility had affected many aspects of her marriage, her relationship with God, even her family and friends. But she had met many incredible women, had found a best friend in Amy, felt closer to Chase than ever for all they'd been through, and most importantly felt closer to God. She had wondered many times what He could possibly be thinking and had reminded herself several times in this second year that He was not doing this to hurt her or Chase. She knew He had a plan and knew best, it was just so hard to see His purposes sometimes. But she reflected on the positive things that had happened because of it and she had felt led to help women who were going through this very thing. She had recently created a blog and shared her thoughts and feelings as well as posted articles written by other women and things she had researched. Not very many people had found her site so far, but several women had told her that she was helping them through the things she was sharing. Jadie knew it was worth it even if she only helped a few people. There was something so wonderful about fellowshipping with other women who understood her core desire and her seeming inability to reach her dreams. She knew God had brought good from this and it made it easier to face the realization that her journey may still have a long way to go yet.

It was November twenty-second, so the exact two year anniversary of their beginning to try was just five days ago. Now

Jadie paced and let her thoughts run wild as her future hung in the balance. She waited for the seemingly millionth time for the dreaded three minutes to pass. Chase was struggling right now with everything and had not wanted her to test today. He told her if she didn't test then he could hold onto the tiny amount of hope he possessed. She told him she wasn't sure she would, but when she'd gotten up that morning she had made up her mind. It was time to find out whether or not this month had worked and stop torturing them both.

For the past couple of months God had gifted Jadie with an overwhelming peace. She was so grateful as she had begun to feel that she couldn't take any more. She had felt like she was trying to walk through waist thick miry clay and God had placed solid ground beneath her feet. Infertility still hurt ... very deeply. She still wondered and hated continuing to wait when her heart felt as though it was bursting with love for her children but with nowhere to direct it. She felt empty at times and hollow and would look down at her arms and wish so badly that it physically hurt that she had a sweet baby in her arms. Tears stung at her eyes at the very thought. So the pain was not gone and she still did fear what they may have yet to face. But the peace that had overcome her felt just like what was mentioned in Philippians 4:7: "And the peace of God, which surpasses all comprehension, will guard your hearts and your minds in Christ Jesus." It was an amazing feeling. She felt like Pilgrim from Pilgrim's Progress and that her burden had been lifted from her back. She felt weightless and free and had more courage to face whatever was in front of them.

Something they'd been waiting for for two years now was answers. She had been waiting and wondering and needed answers at every turn. What was wrong with her? With Chase? Why wasn't it happening? How could they fix it? When would it happen? She found it ironic that the brand of ovulation predictor kits and pregnancy tests she often used was "Answer." She realized that she'd been praying harder than she ever had in her entire life this month and that God was going to give her an answer today. It may not be the one she wanted, but it was an answer all the same. Either they would be pregnant and her prayers would be answered and God would say "Here you go. It's over." or He would say "Wait. It's not time."

Jadie realized she had so much to be thankful for, including the fact that God would answer her today. If the test was negative, she prayed that God would place the same peace on Chase that He had on her and give them both the strength to get through whatever else was ahead of them. She and Chase had talked and were willing to go all the way to IVF and even surrogacy if necessary to have a biological child. They also were open to adoption and once they began going to the specialist again they would have lots of decisions ahead of them depending on what else may be wrong.

It felt insane to Jadie in a way that the answer was forming on a little plastic strip on her bathroom counter. Such a little thing that made such a huge declaration.

Jadie forced herself to sit for a moment on the couch in her living room. She took a deep breath and then closed her eyes. She remembered all they'd been through these past two years. All the pain and heartache. This was their last chance before having to go on to further testing and possibly treatment depending on what the tests revealed. But she once again focused on all the positive God had brought about in her life so far in this journey. She suddenly felt emboldened and knew that as long as she and Chase had God and each other, they could face anything. She prayed and thanked God for all the good He'd brought about in their lives from this experience so far and asked Him to help her accept whatever the test said. Either way, she wanted to look forward to her future with love and hope.

She opened her eyes and smiled from ear to ear. A glance at the clock told her she had allowed four minutes to pass and the test was ready to look at. She stood calmly and walked over to the little hallway that led to their bedroom and turned right towards the bathroom. She looked at her smiling face in the mirror and smiled even wider. She was reminded of Proverbs 31:25b "And she smiles at the future." Yes, that was the woman God had helped grow her to be. She took a quick deep breath and then confidently looked down; ready to face whatever was staring back at her.

A strange feeling bubbled up from her stomach and sent goose bumps up and down her arms. Her mouth dropped open and she picked up the test and held it in better light. In disbelief she stared at the precious symbol she had longed to see for so long . . . years in fact. A positive sign. A beautiful little pink plus sign. She laughed, but it sounded strange and foreign to her own ears. "What? It's positive? I'm pregnant?" she said aloud. "I'm pregnant? I'm pregnant? . . . I . . . I'm pregnant!" Gradually her inflection moved from question to statement. "I can't believe it!" She couldn't take her eyes from the test. "Is this really happening?" She began to pace excitedly around her bedroom. "I'm not dreaming right? It's really happening? Now? I'm going to have a baby?" She laughed and jumped up and down a couple of times and then equally as fast dropped her head and sobs wracked her body. She dropped to her knees and stared at the blurry pink plus sign through her tears. "Thank you, God! Thank you! I just . . . Wow! Thank you so much!" She fell flat on her face and cried and praised God without words since she couldn't coherently form any. She trusted the Holy Spirit to intercede on her behalf and just kept praising Him the best she could. How great and awesome was her God! He would have been if it was negative as well, but she felt overwhelmed by His grace to mercifully end their journey here and bless them with a sweet baby.

A joy that she'd never known filled her and yet she felt strange and in disbelief all at the same time. Instantly fears began to rise to the surface: *What if it's a false positive? What if I'm not really pregnant? Or worse, what if I am but I lose the baby?* "No!" she said aloud. "You will not allow yourself to have these fears. God created this entire universe and He knows and cares about every single bird, so how much more does He care about you

221

and this baby especially when He's the only one who perfectly understands what you've been through? No, Jadie Taylor, you will not allow yourself to go there. God loves you and He has this in His loving hands and you will let it go." She had been extremely stern sounding and now laughed at how ridiculous she would seem to anyone else.

The rest of her day was spent walking on clouds and euphoria as she anxiously awaited Chase getting home. She could never explain her feelings to any one if she tried. But she was on cloud nine and no one could bring her down from there. It was torture waiting to call Amy, but she wanted Chase to be the first one to know. In some ways, it also didn't feel real. She looked at the test many times to reassure herself throughout the day.

By the time four o'clock rolled around (the time Chase had told her this morning he would be coming home), Jadie could hardly contain herself. She'd already put the milk in the cupboard and thrown her brush in the trash can due to her scattered brain and it had taken a few seconds each time for what she'd done to click. She had waited years for this day and hoped she could hold in her excitement long enough to surprise him the way she intended.

Suddenly she heard Chase's truck door slam outside in the driveway and her heart flew in her throat and she jumped off the couch and flew into their bedroom and then back to the door. She tugged at her t-shirt and ran her fingers through her hair to make sure it looked nice and tried to take some steadying breaths as her heart thundered around in her chest. As she watched the door handle turn she took one little step back and used an exorbitant amount of self-restraint to school her features. Chase entered the room and at the sight of him she thought she was going to explode with happiness.

He gave her a tired, lopsided grin. "Hey there! Did you miss me or something, sweety? Waiting for me right by the door?"

She gave a measured smile and said, "I always miss you. How was your day?" and gave him a big hug.

He said on a sigh, "Oh, it was long. How was your day?"

She watched as he removed and hung up his coat and took his gloves off. "Oh, it was good." She drew a steadying breath. "Listen, honey, I have something for you."

He turned to face her and his face was puzzled. "Oh yeah?"

She pulled out a box that looked like a jewelry box from behind her that she had wrapped a blue and pink ribbon around and tied into a bow on the top and held it in front of her so he could see.

"Yeah. You are such a good husband and have been working so hard lately and I thought I'd get you a little something." She smiled and silently jumped up and down inside for sounding so casual about it.

He still looked puzzled, but also pleasantly surprised. "Oh! Well, honey, you didn't have to do that!"

She smiled and twisted her hands anxiously behind her back. "I wanted to. Go ahead and open it." she said and hoped she hadn't sounded too eager.

He smiled up at her and tentatively took off the ribbons and examined the box.

Jadie thought she was going to explode if he didn't hurry up and open it.

He glanced at her one more time and gave her a look like "what could it be?" and then gently opened it.

She watched his eyes grow huge and then his jaw drop open. He stared at it for several seconds and Jadie shifted excitedly and smiled to beat the band. He looked up at her and she had never seen him looked more astonished or shocked in his life. He drug his eyes from his wife's elated face and stared at the test for a few more seconds.

Feeling she'd given him a moment to absorb it, she reached out and took his free hand and said the words she'd wanted to for so long, "I'm pregnant." followed by a slight pause. "You're gonna be a Daddy."

She was still smiling, but suddenly could not speak for the lump that had lodged in her throat. He looked at her with the same shocked expression and said, "Are you serious?" She simply nodded and he carefully closed the lid and pulled her into his arms and held her so tight. Happy tears rolled down Jadie's cheeks and onto Chase's shoulder.

In a hoarse whisper filled with so much depth and emotion he finally said, "Oh, baby. I can't believe it! We're going to have a baby! I love you. I love you so much." He cleared his throat, but she could still tell he was choked up as he said, "Thank you God. Thank you so much!"

They stood that way for several minutes and just rocked slightly as they held each other.

Jadie had never felt more fulfilled or full of joy in her entire life.

❤ ❤ ❤

Jadie and Chase had accomplished a lot since four pm and it was only six o'clock. They had went to the store and bought more pregnancy tests (just to make sure as it still didn't seem real) and went home and watched with joy and elation as each one turned positive nearly instantly. They talked, prayed, and talked some more and were both elated. Chase loved the way she had told him and Jadie was very pleased with herself for pulling off the surprise. After a bit she had called Amy and they had both screamed and jumped up and down as they talked excitedly on the phone. Jadie thought her ears would never stop ringing for how loud her friend had screamed in her ear! Chase just sat on the couch and watched happily as his wife poured out her excitement and good news to her friend. Amy had cried tears of joy and been so elated for her friend and wanted to be filled on every detail of the entire day, including their plans for that night, later. Then Jadie and Chase had spent some time on their phones calling their parents and siblings to all come over for pizza at their house that evening. They were so relieved they were all able to make it despite the late notice. Everyone would start arriving in about fifteen minutes and then she and Chase would make the big announcement. They could hardly wait!

Haden had come home from college for the holidays and shortly after he'd arrived home his mom told him they were invited to Chase and Jadie's house for dinner. He was excited to see his sister and brother-in-law. He missed not seeing them as often now that he had been attending college for a little over a year. Then his mother had non-chalantly added that Chase's family would be joining them as well and Haden's heart nearly fell to his feet. Even though he and Gracie were attending the same school, he didn't see her as much as he would have liked and had still not gotten up the nerve to ask her out or tell her how he felt about her. And now he was standing in his sister's kitchen next to his mother and waiting anxiously for Gracie to arrive.

Jadie and Keira had been trying to include Haden in their conversation, but all he could do was pace nervously and was very distracted. They exchanged a knowing look. Jadie had continued to observe her brother when Gracie was mentioned or if they were around each other ever since his graduation party and she was positive of his affection for her. What she wasn't sure about was why he still hadn't done anything about it. She'd tried to talk to him about it, but he'd always changed the subject and made light of it all. She decided to back off and wait until her brother was ready to talk to her about it. She glanced in the living room and saw Chase talking to her father, Dean, but he seemed more quiet than usual. No doubt trying not to spill the beans, she thought with a giggle. She had liked seeing him so shocked earlier and she enjoyed seeing him more serious and quiet now as well. It was fun for her to watch him be a bit out of character as he was not normally or easily any of those things.

Emily and David were the next to arrive and Gracie had ridden with them. Jadie watched the way her brother got incredibly shy, but she could tell how badly he wanted to speak to her all at the same time. As she observed them throughout the rest of the night, one thing became extremely clear to her. Her brother did not have a crush, was not infatuated, and was not smitten.

He was in love. It touched her very much and she thought they would make a wonderful match. Now she just had to stick to her resolve to stay out of the situation until Haden invited her in.

Not long after Emily, David, and Gracie had arrived, Chase's brother Finn and his wife Sarah arrived with their little boy Charlie and their seven month old daughter, Lily. For the first time Jadie was able to kiss her sweet nephew and niece without any sadness or longing and only happiness to see them along with the joy that she too would have a child of her own. It was a wonderful feeling!

Once every one had mingled a bit, Chase and Finn went to get the pizzas and when they got back every one gathered around the kitchen for Chase to pray. He grinned at Jadie and took her hand. "We're happy you're all here with us tonight. It's nice to have the family together. But more than just having a night of fun and pizza, we have something we'd like to say." He squeezed her hand and they smiled at each other and then said in unison, "We're going to have a baby!" in a very excited tone. The room burst forth with cheers, congratulations, exclamations of happiness, and hugs all around. Chase had even hidden the video camera next to the toaster at an angle that caught every one before hand and had sneakily turned it on before the announcement was made. Jadie was glad they'd always have this moment on video, but she knew she didn't need it. She would never forget this night as long as she lived.

The rest of the evening was filled with eating pizza, talking about the baby, playing cards, laughing, and visiting until late. Jadie was glad Haden even had a chance to sneak Gracie outside for a quick walk in the brisk evening air.

After every one had gone home after midnight and Chase had helped her clean up the kitchen, they snuggled together in their nice warm bed and talked more about their baby. They prayed together and finally started trying to go to sleep after one a.m. Jadie snuggled a little closer to Chase and smiled against her pillow and released a content and happy sigh. Life was great and God was so good.

Chapter 24

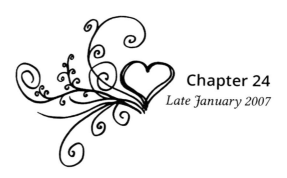

Chapter 24
Late January 2007

Amy smiled as she watched the girls play on the floor of her living room. Maddie was happily kicking, playing, and cooing as she played on her floor gym and Meg was talking to her in sweet voices in between playing with her toys next to her. They both were so beautiful inside and out and Amy felt her heart swell with a love she'd never known as she watched them. The way it did multiple times a day.

Poor Jadie's e-mail must have been tired by now from all the pictures she had sent her of the girls. She also updated Jadie regularly on all the cute things they were doing, their personalities, and how they were adjusting. Amy remembered vividly just a few months ago wanting to remove any of the fear and vulnerability from the little sweethearts' faces. Most traces of that were gone now and they were completely comfortable with Jake and Amy. In fact, just yesterday, Meg had called Amy "momma" and Amy had dropped to her knees and hugged the little girl so she wouldn't see the tears in her eyes. She'd never heard a sweeter sound in all the world and she prayed she always would get that special title from both of the little beauties before her.

Just a few weeks ago she and Jake had received news that the biological mother's rights had been terminated. She apparently had not only not been making attempts to meet the requirements set for her by the court, but had also apparently broken some crucial requirement of her parole. The judge had had enough and terminated her rights immediately. The woman's family had been contacted and none of them wanted custody. And since they had been with Jake and Amy almost from the day they had been removed from their mother and things were going so well, they had been given the green light to proceed with the adoption process. Amy and Jake couldn't have been more thrilled! Although they did pray for the girls' mother each night and that God would keep her safe and work in her life. But their case worker had assured them that other than the paperwork and formalities and waiting until things were official, the girls were as good as their's. Amy felt overwhelmed by the blessing of it all. Things had moved ahead so much sooner than she even expected and now she and Jake were adopting their two precious girls. It was as if God had hand-chosen them for she and Jake and Amy couldn't have been more grateful.

They had all had a beautiful Christmas. Both Amy and Jake's families had been very supportive of their decision to pursue foster care and they had shown love and acceptance of the girls while also being so careful to not smother or overwhelm them. Amy appreciated their sensitivity and knew all the members of their families had also come to adore their girls as they did. So it had made for a beautiful holiday and Amy also was so glad to be moving into a new year and her new future as a family of four. She got goose bumps just thinking of themselves that way, but they truly felt like a family.

Jadie couldn't have been more thrilled about the news! Or Chase for that matter. When Amy had called to tell her they were proceeding with the adoption, Jadie had put the phone on speaker and Chase had whooped and hollered and carried on for a full minute. Amy had put the phone on speaker so Jake could hear and it was fun to watch her husband belly laugh as he didn't all that often being a more somber man. Amy had laughed until tears nearly rolled down her cheeks from Jadie going from crying and blubbering to squealing in delight all while laughing at her husband for his reaction as well. It was a wonderful memory that Amy knew she would always cherish.

The front door opened and shut and Amy was interrupted from her musings. Her husband was home! He smiled hugely, as he did more often these days, as he walked into the living room. She stood and gave him a hug and kiss and they exchanged greetings and "I love you's" and then he went directly to the floor to play with the girls. Meg instantly crawled into his lap and began holding up all of her toys for him to see, which he carefully inspected as he talked to her about each one in a sweet voice. He leaned down and kissed Maddie's cheek and she smiled happily and began kicking like crazy in her excitement to see him. He laughed and tickled her and played peek-a-boo until both girls were giggling outright. Amy grabbed her camera, which she always had handy now, and snapped a couple of shots and then joined her husband on the floor. He placed an arm around her and kissed her temple while still holding Meg on the other side. Amy smiled contentedly up at him and they just looked at each other. No words were needed. Their happiness was complete. They looked at each other tenderly for quite awhile and with more love in their eyes than ever, just smiling to beat the band. Meg began pulling on Jake's shirt to get his attention, so they started playing with the girls.

After a couple of minutes, Jake placed Meg in Amy's lap and put Maddie in his own. He grabbed the camera sitting next to Amy and leaned close to her and held it out in front of them. They both smiled with all the joy that filled their hearts as Jake snapped the picture. Amy looked at it on the little digital screen and knew that it was one for the mantle. She, Jake, and their precious little girls. Her beautiful little family.

❤ ❤ ❤

Jadie's heart beat fast in anticipation as the nurse placed the warm gel on her belly. Any moment now she was going to see their baby for the second time on ultrasound and she could hardly wait. She stared at the screen and squeezed Chase's hand. As the nurse placed the wand on Jadie's belly, the picture of their little peanut instantly filled the screen. Jadie's eyes filled with tears as she looked at the beautiful little baby . . . her baby . . . their baby.

Jadie marveled at God's wondrous creation as she saw all the perfect little limbs, sweet profile, and adorable hands and feet as their baby squirmed around inside of her. She glanced at Chase and he too had tears in his eyes and a big smile plastered on his face. He looked at her, his eyes so full of love it nearly took Jadie's breath. She knew it was for her and the baby and she felt blessed to have such a wonderful husband and knew he was going to be an amazing daddy. He was already very protective of her and the baby which Jadie found both endearing and sweet.

She looked back to the screen and in some ways still couldn't believe this was happening. That she had a precious baby growing inside of her and was finally a mother. She and Chase had a baby and she felt like the most blessed and happiest girl alive.

She had been sick for a couple of weeks, but other than that felt pretty good other than being tired a lot. She had to take some time off work due to the fact that she was high risk for the first four months and couldn't be on her feet like she would be all day at the flower shop. But her boss was very understanding and she would be returning to work once the "high risk" label was removed. Jadie would take the prometrium until that time to make sure her body had enough progesterone to maintain her pregnancy. Other than the sickness, Jadie had adored being pregnant. It was the most amazing thing to her and something she never knew if she would get to experience. She thought back to how she used to be agitated when women would complain about being pregnant and used to tease that she would be laughing while throwing up if she ever got pregnant. She chuckled to herself now knowing that wasn't really how it had turned out. But still, she appreciated and cherished her pregnancy very much!

She and Amy had both remained on the TTC group offering support to those who were still trying. Jadie figured she would stay on for awhile longer, but eventually leave. That part of her journey was over, although the pain and sadness were still so recent and real to her. She no longer felt the pain, but she remembered it well. She knew her heart would always bear the scars of infertility and although it sounded strange, she felt proud to be counted among those who had experienced it and that she and Chase had survived it somehow.

She decided to reminisce later and continued to watch her baby with intense joy for the remainder of the ultrasound. It seemed it was over much too soon, but she and Chase fussed over the pictures for several minutes in the parking lot before heading on their way.

They stopped at a big baby store and walked hand-in-hand and did something Jadie had only ever dreamed about: they started their registry for their baby. It was something Jadie had only ever imagined and she felt like she was walking on a cloud as she and Chase wandered through the store and dreamed and planned for their baby. She used to somewhat avoid the baby section of stores because it made her sad and was yet another painful reminder of what she didn't and may never have. So to walk the store now with her sweet husband and look for things their precious baby would use filled Jadie with such an intense joy she thought she may explode! She and Chase talked excitedly about the baby as they walked through the store and they expressed many times how much God had blessed them and how He had brought them through. It had been hard to feel in the dark for so long and they couldn't see the light at the end of the tunnel, but God had. He had His plans and purposes for them, and as the verse they cherished said: not to harm them, and now look at them. They were going to be a little family. Jadie placed her hand on her little baby bump and felt the joy radiate through her entire body. Chase placed his hand over her's and leaned his head on her's. "I love you both so much."

She smiled and replied with all the love she felt in her heart, "Me too, Chase. You have no idea how much."

♥ ♥ ♥

Amy had just cleaned up from dinner and peeked in at her husband rocking both girls in his lap in the recliner. Maddie had already dropped off and Meg was heading there. Amy smiled warmly as she dried her hands on her dishtowel and then hung it up to dry. Just then the phone rang and she grabbed it quickly so it didn't disturb her little family.

"Hey, Amy! Is this a bad time?"

She kept her voice low. "Not at all, Jadie! I'm glad you called. Jake is snuggling the girls and I think all three of them are on their way out."

"Awww, that's so precious! You'll have to send me a picture."

"You know me! I already took one, so I will!"

They shared a laugh.

"So, I wanted to call and update you about my ultrasound."

"That's right! I was going to check my e-mail before bed and see if you had sent me any pictures."

"I will have to do that tomorrow! I haven't had a chance to scan them into my computer yet. Oh Amy, it was amazing! The baby is just so beautiful and precious."

"I'm sure! I wish I could go to an appointment with you."

"Aww, me too! I will be sure to get you the pictures ASAP though."

They talked for a few more minutes about the ultrasound, Chase and Jadie registering, and all the cute things Meg and Maddie had done that day, including their lively bath earlier.

Then Jadie grew serious and said, "Amy, I just want to thank you."

"For what?" Amy asked, genuinely not knowing what her friend was referring to.

"For being my friend. I don't know what I would have done

the last two years without you."

The sincerity in her friend's voice warmed Amy's heart and she could tell her friend was choked up as well. "Oh Jadie. I feel the same way! You helped get me through the toughest part of our infertility journey. I know God brought us together to help one another."

"He certainly did! He really knew what He was doing all along even though I couldn't see it. Thank you for reminding me of that along the way and just encouraging me in Him through all this."

"His plan certainly turned out great for both of us. And you're welcome. You did the same for me!"

"Yeah, but you're just so much stronger than me. You went through so much more and handled it with so much strength and faith. I just look up to you so much!"

"Aww, thank you. I wouldn't say I'm stronger than you, I think you did great too. And trust me, I needed your support just as much as you needed mine."

"Thanks." Jadie sighed loudly. "I just feel glad that it's all behind us and we are in such a beautiful season now. But at the same time, I'm grateful for what it taught me, how it brought me closer to God, closer to Chase, and brought me my best friend. I wouldn't change it, ya know?"

Amy felt her throat grow tight. "I absolutely do and feel the exact same way as you about all of it. Thank you for being my friend too, Jadie. I know we will always stay friends too, this is just the beginning!"

"You're right and that's another amazing blessing that came out of all of this. I'm just so so happy for all of us, but so heartbroken for those who are still going through it."

Amy felt the weight in her heart that she felt for every one anywhere who was going through that. "I know just what you mean. We will have to keep reminding each other to be praying for everyone and maybe we can even find a way to be a support to other women somehow. Maybe start our own group or website or something."

Jadie gasped. "That sounds amazing! We totally should! We'll talk more later, but I'm so excited now!"

Amy laughed at her friends' enthusiasm.

"Well, I'll let you get your little family to bed and I'm pretty tired from today, so I think Chase and I are going to turn in early."

"Okay, we'll talk soon."

"Yes. Good night, Amy." Jadie's voice reflected how true it was as she said, "I love you, friend."

Amy smiled and felt even happier, if that was possible. "Good night, sweet Jadie. I love you too."

Epilogue

Two-and-a-Half Years Later
June 2009

Jadie reached back and tightened her ponytail by dividing it into two sections between her fingers and pulling them away from each other. She adjusted her seat belt and stared wide-eyed out the window. She blew all the air out of her lungs and one of her legs bounced up and down uncontrollably. Chase stole a glance and smiled at her before diverting his gaze back to the road in front of them. "Jadie, honey," He said in a sweet voice, "Just relax. You're not nervous are you? I mean, you girls have been friends for years now!" She smiled slightly and glanced at him with those beautiful green eyes that he loved looking into so much. He forced his eyes back to the road. She sighed before replying, "No, I'm not nervous. Just anxious, I guess. You know, it's the first time we'll have met each other in person. I know we are close and care deeply for each other, but it's just . . . "

"The unknown?" He completed for her.

"Exactly!" she said a little louder than she'd intended to. She cleared her throat and continued more calmly, "You know how I am meeting people for the first time. But this time it's just so much more important than ever before. I mean, I know she'll like me. I know she does already." She laughed somewhat awkwardly.

He smiled again. "You're just really excited about this aren't you, honey? You guys have shared so much over the years. Your bond goes so deep. And it's just . . . a different kind of relationship. It's always been online or on the phone. And sure, you guys have heard each other's voices, but it's not the same as meeting in person and interacting with each other."

She smiled at him. "I love the way you understand me. I think that's it." Her eyes seemed trained on everything that was whizzing past them outside the window. "I'm so excited to see her. But I guess I do feel a tad bit nervous as well. I know I shouldn't, it's just . . . there."

He reached across the small distance between him and gently took her hand in his. "I understand, baby. But don't worry. You have always said how it seems like you two have known each other all of your life. I'm sure it will feel completely natural when you are together."

"You're right, I'm sure it will."

Chase was glad her voice had sounded more relaxed during that statement. He also noticed her leg had stopped bouncing during their conversation. He checked his rear view mirror and smiled. He was so excited for them to meet in person finally. He even had to admit he was excited about meeting Amy and Jake. He felt like he knew them fairly well himself, through Jadie. This would be a wonderful experience for all of them. He squeezed Jadie's hand beside him. They would be there soon.

♥ ♥ ♥

Amy wiped at the picnic table again trying to remove the dirt that seem practically imbedded into the wood. She had that adorable frown on her face like she always did when her mind was working and she was stubbornly trying to fix something. Jake smiled widely, but tried to hide it. She wanted everything to be perfect when Jadie and Chase arrived. They had been waiting at the park now for about twenty minutes. Already Amy had the tablecloth on the table and the contents of her picnic basket emptied. She had also set the two liters of soda pop up and had the cups, plates, and napkins all ready to go. The cameras were out and were ready to be used. The tablecloth didn't quite reach to the ends of the table and that's why she was in a little tizzy now. He stood up from his place on the bench of the picnic table next to the one she was at and walked over to her. He didn't hesitate, but just took her in his arms. "Honey, the table looks great. Don't worry about it." He felt her relax slightly in his arms.

Amy smiled up at the man she loved so dearly. She loved how that deep voice of his just melted her heart every time and how well he understood her and always knew just what to do to make her feel better. She felt slightly silly for the way she'd been acting all day, but she was so excited, anxious, and slightly nervous she could hardly stand it. Did Jadie feel the same way?

They had set up this meeting nearly two months prior when they found out they were both going to be traveling the same highway the same week to go on their family vacations. They had rearranged their schedules just slightly and scoured over detailed maps until they agreed on a recreational stop that they both would be passing.

Amy looked up at Jake, who was still holding her, and said, "You don't suppose they got lost do you?"

He hugged her just a little tighter and replied, "No, honey. We were early, remember? They'll be here in no time. You'll see." He finished this by adding one of his most confident smiles.

"You're right. They'll be here soon."

Jake released her and Amy began to straighten and fuss a bit more, but not with the passion she had a moment ago. Jake shook his head and wondered if Chase had been dealing with this same thing and had the same conversation with Jadie that he had had with Amy earlier this morning. He chuckled to himself. This was all fine by him. He knew these girls were more than ready to meet each other. Especially after all they had been through together.

♥ ♥ ♥

Jadie stared intently at the print out of the map quest map she held in her hand. "Okay, yeah, it's about a mile up here on the right." She fidgeted in her seat. How long she had waited for this day! She was growing more and more giddy by the moment. It seemed like no time and Chase turned his blinker on. She felt her pulse quicken. This was it! They wove down and around a few curves and it was nice to actually be near the trees instead of just see them off to the side of the bare road. She kept craning her neck this way and that trying to see if she could see the Whitley family yet. Finally she saw in the distance a tall, dark haired man sitting on the seat of a picnic table and a woman with hair like Amy's wearing a pink T-shirt and jeans.

"That's them!" she said in a high pitch voice and the hugest smile on her face.

Chase smiled. "Sure is. Try to stay in your seat until I can get the car parked."

He laughed heartily after saying this because Jadie was literally bouncing up and down in her seat.

By the time they pulled into the space, they were maybe fifteen feet from the couple. Jadie felt her throat grow tight when she saw two adorable little girls running around the table and a baby in a stroller that was parked very close to where Jake sat. One little girl had brown hair that was a few inches past her shoulders and the older one had long blonde hair. They had very different faces, but you could tell they were sisters. They both wore adorable sundresses and white tennis shoes. She of course had seen the girls at times in pictures, but she hadn't seen recent ones in awhile and to see them in person was different entirely. Jadie unfastened her seat belt and climbed slowly out of the car. She had both feet on the ground, but just stood unmoving for a moment hanging onto the top of the door with one hand, watching the happy scene unfold before her. Jake smiled at her and she suddenly realized her mouth was gaping open. She flashed him a quick smile and then quickly turned her gaze to Amy, whom up until now, had had her back to her and was bending over picking something up. She sat it on the table, straightened, and slowly turned as she did so. Tears instantly misted her eyes as she locked eyes with Jadie. Jadie smiled through tears of her own and tried not to choke on a sob. She slammed her car door shut and jogged over to Amy, whose arms were open wide before Jadie even reached her.

The women embraced and both cried. Neither one felt one bit awkward, only elated to finally meet one another after all the things they had been through together, the miles that had separated them, and the years of never seeing each other in person. Jadie thought that this was even better than she imagined and how wonderful it felt to hug the woman who had been her pillar, her rock, her sympathizer, and her closest friend. Amy was thinking how wonderful it felt to hug the sweetest woman she'd ever known after wanting to be able to countless times over the years. Both of them felt so natural and so completely happy. The tears streamed down their faces as the hug continued and they also talked excitedly to one another and laughed from time to time. Their bond was so deep and it was obvious by the way they carried on that way for over five minutes. The men had smiled at each other, shook hands, and took the liberty of introducing themselves quietly while standing back a bit to give the women this moment. Both men felt very happy and proud of their wives. The women finally pulled apart and were able to meet their friends' husbands as well. Jadie gave Jake a quick hug and Amy shook Chase's hand, who pulled her into a one armed hug, causing her to laugh.

They all visited for just a moment and Jadie's eyes had been wandering to the stroller that was only three or so feet away from her. Amy suddenly went serious and glanced down and noticed the adorable toddler who was shyly smiling at her while hanging onto her daddy's pointer and middle finger with a near death grip. Jadie followed her gaze and smiled broadly. She kneeled down and her daughter released her daddy's hand and walked over to her side. Jadie put her arm around her and smiled up at Amy who had begun to kneel down in front of her.

Jadie said sweetly, and with much pride, "There is someone very important I want you to meet. This is my daughter, Lizabeth."

Amy's eyes had once again misted with tears and she held her hand out to her friend's adorable little girl. She was slightly small for being a little under two years old and had a beautiful little face that looked mostly like Jadie, but had touches of Chase as well. She had gotten her blonde hair from Chase and also had his ears. But the big green eyes, freckles, and most of her facial structure were all from her momma.

Jadie put her cheek against her toddler's head and said, "This is your Aunt Amy that we talk about every day and I show you her picture." The little girls' smile widened and to both women's surprise she suddenly ran the short distance to Amy and threw her arms around her neck. Amy's eyes slid shut as she hugged the child and a few tears slid down her cheeks. A few slid down Jadie's as well. Amy was so glad God had given Jadie her miracle . . . her precious Lizzy. It was one of the most amazing feelings in the world to hold her friend's child who was truly a gift from God. She remembered well when Jadie had called her the day after Lizabeth was born to tell her all about the birth. When Jadie had told Amy the baby's weight and length, she had paused for a moment and her voice was soft with feeling as she said, "We named her Lizabeth," followed by another short pause, ". . . after you, Amy." She had teared up then and it made a couple more tears slide down her cheeks now. Amy's middle name was "Elizabeth." The pronunciation of Lizabeth's name was how it would sound to just cut the "E" at the beginning out. Amy flashed back to the present and forced herself to release little Lizzy.

Once Lizzy went back to her dad and Jadie and Amy had stood, Jadie gently took Amy's hand and placed it on her slightly swollen tummy.

"And this is little no name baby" and all four adults laughed.

Amy asked, "You are fourteen weeks now, aren't you Jadie?"

Jadie smiled broadly and said, "Yes. I feel great and we are just so excited."

Jake chimed in with a question of his own. "Do you guys think it's a girl or a boy?"

Jadie had went to Chase's side and they had their arms around each other and both smiled widely. "A boy" they said in unison causing Amy and Jake to laugh again.

"Speaking of boys," Amy said as she began walking towards the stroller, "here is our little guy." The others had followed and Jadie felt her heart beat harder as they drew closer to the stroller. Amy had not allowed her to see pictures of him since they had gotten him three months ago and already knew by then they'd probably be seeing each other that summer. Jadie finally peered in and gasped softly when she saw the adorable, alert seven-month-old baby staring back at her. He had dark brown hair, bright blue eyes, and the roundest face and was beyond precious. While Amy got him out so Jadie could hold him, Jake had called the girls over. Both parents grinned with pride as they introduced Meg, Maddie, and Matthew. Jadie hugged both sweet little girls before holding Matthew. Both she and Chase kept saying how beautiful they all were.

"I can't believe the girls are four and three already!" Jadie commented.

Amy nodded. "I know what you mean. Meg will be starting kindergarten this fall already."

Jadie shook her head in disbelief.

Momentary silence fell over the group and Jadie felt that it was so surreal that she was really with her friend and had met her children. Little did she know her friend was having similar thoughts. They shared a look with each other that needed no words. Jadie felt her throat grow thick and said a quick prayer. *We both got our miracles. In different ways, but we both have our precious children. Thank you, God.*

♥ ♥ ♥

Once they had sat and ate lunch together and all visited and had plenty of laughs, the men took the kids off a ways to play so the women could have some time to visit. Jadie asked Amy to fill her in on the adoption of Matthew since it was private this time instead of through the state. Amy proceeded to share the differences between the two, more about the whole process, and how although she and Jake would consider adoption again in the future whether through the state or private, that they preferred private.

"But, we are open to whatever the Lord has planned for us," she closed with.

Jadie nodded. "I know you already know this, but Chase and I have been talking more and more about adoption lately. I think that we want to try for one more, but we'd also like to adopt one. Pray for us about that, would you?"

Amy's smile had nearly stretched across her face while Jadie had been talking. She slid her hand over Jadie's and gave it a quick squeeze. "Always. I'm more than thrilled for you guys. I can't wait to see what God will do!"

Jadie flashed her friend one of her sweetest smiles.

Amy decided to change the subject. "Jadie? Will you tell me again? How it felt to hold Lizzy in your arms for the first time."

Jadie knew from their many discussions that Amy was completely at peace with the fact that she would never carry her own children, but still Jadie's heart constricted and she had to ask, "Are you sure Amy? That you want to hear about this, I mean?"

"Absolutely. I appreciate you being concerned for me, Jadie, but I promise it won't hurt me. Maybe a few years ago it still may have stung a bit even though I was at peace with God's will for us in this. But not anymore."

Jadie felt relief spread through her at the confidence in her friends' voice and face.

Amy continued, "I received my miracles. Three of them. And they are no less mine because I didn't carry them. I don't feel less of a mother. And I know you don't think that, but I'm just letting you know. It doesn't hurt me anymore that I won't ever have that first moment in that hospital bed. Meeting my children for the first time was still one of the best moments in my life besides accepting the Lord as my Savior and my wedding day with Jake. And it's how God intended it to be for us and I just feel . . . I don't know. Very happy and complete."

She smiled and added with a wink, "And I didn't even have to go through labor and delivery to get my kids which is a perk."

Jadie laughed and then told her friend that she understood

and how happy she was for her, meaning every word with her whole heart.

Then she proceeded to answer Amy's question. "It's hard to put into words really. When they held her up so I could see her, it felt as though I had waited an entire lifetime to get to that moment. And the few inches the doctor had to raise her for me to see felt like ten minutes. And when I finally did see her, I'd never seen anything more beautiful in my entire life. There she was . . . my child. Something I hadn't been sure would ever happen for me had. Her little eyes were blinking and looking around and she hardly cried. It was like a sign or something that no one needed to be upset in that moment." She chuckled. "I know that sounds ridiculous, but that's just how I felt at the time. She was perfect. Absolutely perfect." Amy noticed Jadie's eyes had taken on a distant look and she was staring at a spot in the grass unblinking. She knew her friend was reliving every moment and would never forget it as long as she lived. "Me and Chase and in one tiny little person. It's the most amazing thing!"

Amy smiled. "Indeed!"

There was a comfortable silence and then Amy shared something with her friend.

"You know, I was thinking just now when I said I felt happy and complete."

Jadie had turned to face Amy and was listening intently.

"I know people who adopt, but it doesn't take away their desire for biological children. I can completely see that, but I guess I'm glad I still don't feel that desire. I think that would be so hard to still want that as much as we used to, but to know that would never be a possibility for us. I used to pray that if God didn't want me to have biological children that He'd take that desire away. I haven't thought about it in a long time, but I guess He did! I guess I just feel lucky to not have to still have that pain. I pray for those who adopt yet still have that desire all the time. I just think it would be so difficult."

Jadie solemnly nodded. "There are just so many aspects to

infertility aren't there? I still hurt for all those who go through it and pray for them often."

Amy nodded as well and then wanted to lighten the mood, so she smiled and said, "Well, that's the best thing we can do. But you know what? I think now we need dessert!"

Jadie was not even remotely expecting that comment nor her friends' silly and serious tone and tipped her head back and her laughter rang out in the air.

♥ ♥ ♥

Jake and Chase had both been getting plenty of video footage of the kids playing together, the women visiting, and other things they had done throughout the day as a group. They had also brought their tri-pod and had gotten all different combinations of pictures of the group: just the kids, just the adults, just the two women, family shots, and a few of them all together. Chase felt as though they had been at a family reunion all day. A few minutes earlier he had heard Jadie mention that they only had about two hours left together before it was time to go. His heart had clenched at the sadness in her voice. He knew she would probably cry as they drove away knowing she would be even more attached to her friend, but not able to see her again for quite some time. But already today they had made plans to go visit Amy and Jake at their home in Wyoming the next summer for their family vacation. He knew that Jadie and Amy would be lifelong friends.

He came out of his musing and looked at Jake who was seated beside him at a picnic table, their legs facing away from the table. The men were watching the children play not far in front of them. Jake looked back and flashed him a big smile. "Can you believe that we both have families now?"

Chase smiled and shook his head, "It's amazing. There were times I thought it may never happen."

Jake looked solemn and nodded his agreement. "I'm so glad it's behind us now. I do think it made us stronger as people, and as a couple, for that matter. I'll always remember the pain of it though."

He stretched his arm out, palm up and moved his hand around in the direction of the children playing in front of them. "It makes all this that much sweeter, you know?"

Chase sighed contentedly and said, "It sure does."

The men sat together for a few more minutes with their thoughts before Jake said, "You wanna play another game of frizz-bee?"

Chase smiled. "Sounds great."

♥ ♥ ♥

Jadie and Amy continued to watch their families play, including their husbands, while they talked. They both sat with their legs facing away from the picnic table, their elbows resting on the table portion much the way the men had been doing not long ago. The sun was quickly sinking beneath the trees behind them. "Amy? I know we've talked about this before, but don't you feel like your marriage is even stronger and I don't know ... sweeter than before?"

Amy nodded. "Absolutely. There were times it was so hard, but God got us through. I definitely feel like we're closer now than we've ever been."

"I feel the same way about Chase and I. Just when I think I can't love him anymore, I continue to every day. Like just now, watching him play with our kids and the way he scoops Lizzy up now and then and makes her giggle. It never stops just absolutely melting my heart. I can't remember how many times I wished so badly to see that very thing." Her heart constricted for a moment just remembering that pain. Though she now felt whole, she knew her heart would always bear the scars of what they'd been through.

Amy nodded again. "Yes. Seeing your husband with your children is definitely one of the sweetest things you'll ever see."

They went on to talk about their first impressions of each

other and their friendship over the years. They talked about hard times, happy things they had experienced, and funny stories and experiences.

"I'm so glad that God brought us into each other's lives" Jadie said solemnly once they had gotten done laughing from all their stories.

Amy smiled. "I couldn't agree more, Jadie. Isn't it a neat thought that we'll not only be friends the rest of our lives here on earth, but we'll also spend eternity together?"

It was nearly dark and Jadie watched their husbands and children trying to catch the lightning bugs. "Wow, I hadn't really thought about that. What an amazing thing."

Jadie stood and Amy did the same.

Amy playfully bumped elbows with Jadie and smiled at her. "We have come a long way, haven't we?"

Jadie looked again at the scene before her and knew exactly what Amy meant. "Yes, we have. The beginnings of wondering what was wrong, the stress, the wonder, the unanswered questions, going through different phases emotionally, the doctors visits and trying things out, the waiting and waiting . . . and waiting. And finally . . . " Despite the light mood, her throat grew thick from the tears that threatened to come. She took a breath and lovingly placed her hand on her slightly rounded stomach. "Finally, we got our miracles."

Amy put her arm around her. "Yes, and what a long road here it was. We've had quite the journey."

Jadie slipped her arm around Amy's waist. "Yeah, we sure have. I'm just glad I had my husband, you, and most importantly God to get me through it."

Amy smiled affectionately at her as happy tears glistened in her eyes. "Amen to that sister!"

They both laughed.

"You know what?" Jadie asked.

"What?" Amy replied, her arm still around Jadie's shoulders.

"Even though our journeys were different, we both got our

miracles. But there was one big thing we had in common even before either of us knew what we would face. And both of us had it fulfilled."

"What's that?"

The most peaceful expression crossed Jadie's face and her heart was so full of love for all those around her. She was so grateful for all God had done in her life. She looked at Amy and smiled. "The heart of a mother."

Amy smiled back. It was so true.

A Word From the Author

I feel I'm just overflowing with things I want to say about infertility and all that can be involved, even though I feel the story in this book covers a lot of those issues! First I do want to say that all of the characters in this book are completely fictional and are not based on any one I know. Obviously their experiences are shaped from something I have experienced personally, have learned from all of my friends who have gone through this or the girls from my TTC group, or at least something I can imagine or a combination of these things.

I want to say as well that I am certainly no Doctor! I based what the girls in this story went through (test, medication, and treatment wise) on what other women had to say about their experiences and through Internet research. But I am not endorsing any particular drug or method. If you are facing any kind of issue where you may need medication for TTC, hormonal issues, or something similar; please speak to your Doctor, your family, and do some research of your own and of course pray, and go from there. This is a fictional story but I did want it to be accurate and specific, so certain things are based on what other women have been through, but that doesn't mean I am recommending any certain type of medication, etc.

I think infertility is often an overlooked issue. Most people don't think about it unless they end up facing this challenge themselves. That is how it was for my husband and I, anyways. It's one of those things that you think will never happen to you. But I hope this book brings some education to my readers about infertility, may help someone who is beginning to realize something "isn't right," help encourage, give hope, and heal the hearts of those who have gone/are going through it, and help develop more compassion and understanding in those who have not gone through it.

When I began working on this book, the most common statistic I found was that one in ten couples experienced infertility. By the time I finished this book, the more common statistic was one in eight couples. While the fact that many couples are waiting until later in life certainly affects that statistic to a degree, there are still many things that are unknown as to why it is so common. A misconception is that infertility is usually a "woman's issue," when in fact about one-third of the time it is the female, one-third of the time it is the male, and one-third of the time it is both or is unexplained. Infertility also is a recognized disease (automatic diagnosis after one year of unprotected sex) by The American Society for Reproductive Medicine (ASRM) and the American College of Obstetricians and Gynecologists (ACOG) and the World Health Organization (WHO). It is the result of one or both partners' reproductive systems not working correctly (and sadly is sometimes even unexplained) and is also defined as the inability to carry a pregnancy all the way to birth. But it is a physical issue and if you research it, you will find that it is not caused by stress (probably the biggest misconception there is about infertility). An excellent resource for both those who have gone through infertility or those who want to know more about it is RESOLVE: The National Infertility Association. They have so much information for couples struggling with infertility and also for people who are trying to educate themselves or know someone with infertility. They also have information on local support groups and so on. Their website is: *www.resolve.org*.

The most important issues I wanted to shine out in this book are: the isolation that someone feels as they are going through this, how much having the support of someone who is going through what you are can help, for someone who is going through it to not feel alone, for those who have not gone through it to understand it from people who go through it's perspective, and just how difficult it is in general. I hope that I have accomplished my goal with this book of opening people's eyes to what infertility is really like and have shown, at least to a degree, what we (who have gone or are going through infertility) feel and experience. I feel like I was only able to touch on it even though the whole book is about it. Many people who go through infertility suffer for many more years and go through much more testing and treatment than the characters in this book did. I only just scratched the surface of what all people can go through with this disease. I also realize I'm a new writer and I have a lot of learning and improvement ahead of me, but I pray that the story touched every one the way I hoped it would.

I hope I did all the women and couples who go through this justice since they often don't have the chance to fully express themselves. Many of us who suffer with infertility do so silently. Not only does it seem to be an overlooked issue, but one that is very misunderstood. Of course it also feels private in nature which causes people to keep it to themselves. I hope and pray I did well in explaining the emotions and feelings and insane ups and downs these couples go through on their journeys. People who go through this will always carry a special place in my heart. My prayers are with the many couples experiencing infertility.

Something I recommend if you are struggling at all emotionally or mentally with the whole trying to conceive process is to get support. I know that this helped me immensely. Finding women (or men) who are going through the same thing as you is extremely comforting. They will understand the stress, the wondering, the strain it can cause, the wondering if you're going crazy and are just imagining symptoms or if they are really there, and why you think you will just not be able to bear it any longer if you hear one more person tell you "Just relax, and it will happen" or "being stressed out is going to hinder you even more from getting pregnant." There are websites, forums, groups, you name it of women out there going through the same thing. It's an excellent place to vent and be understood and encourage one another. Also, many women on those groups have a lot of knowledge and you may even find someone in your exact circumstance who can give you advice. Once I felt like something may not be right, I joined a yahoo group for TTC (trying to conceive) women and I was blown away by the support, understanding, suggestions, and knowledge of the women on that group. It helped me immensely. And it was also ultimately what led me to discover what was going on with my body. I also decided to open up and share with my group of online friends about my frustrations only to find that at least four of my friends had also experienced infertility! So they were an amazing help to me also. Experiencing infertility can feel extremely isolating, so know that there are options out there for you if you don't know any one personally who is going through it.

My advice to you if you know someone who is going through infertility would be:

- Don't tell them to relax, take a vacation, or adopt and then they will get pregnant. This not only invalidates their pain, but makes it seem as if it is their fault or that these things will "cure" them (which they well know that it won't).
- Let them know that you're praying for them.
- Just be a listening ear. Let them know you care. You have no idea how much this will help them!
- If you do say something that hurts them and they get brave enough to tell you that, please don't say it again.
- Don't pretend you know what God is doing by telling them that maybe He doesn't want them to be parents or that they're not meant to be parents.
- Try to be understanding if they don't want to attend baby showers or constantly be around pregnant women and the like. This is a constant reminder of what they are missing. They are in deep emotional turmoil and may need space from these things at times.
- If you are unsure about what to say, don't say anything. Just be there for them and pray for them.

♥ ♥ ♥

Sharing my story . . .

Originally I felt that I would keep my difficulty in this area to myself. First because it is so personal and secondly probably partially because of pride. I didn't want the questions or for people to feel like there was something "wrong" with me. When I decided to write this book, I knew I would share my story and that it wouldn't remain private anymore. I want other women to feel emboldened as well to share their stories with others whether to help them, encourage them, or just because they need someone to talk to. And I wanted to share my story in case it would help even just one person know that they are not alone. While the character of Jadie in this book is not based on me personally and her story is fictional, much of what she experiences with her infertility issues is based on my personal experiences. So as you read this book and see what issues arise with Jadie, you will in many instances see what has happened to me. Every scene with Jadie is not necessarily based on my own experience, but her reason for not being able to conceive without medical help and the treatment she goes through and some of her feelings are based on me.

My husband and I began trying in August of 2007 much the same way I had Chase and Jadie start out. We had carefully and prayerfully thought about what time would be best for us. We had also waited awhile as we wanted to be married for 4-5 years before starting a family. So we sat on our bed and read our Bible together, prayed, and talked and dreamed about our future with children. Month after month went by and I tried to stay positive, but began to get worried some. I joined a yahoo group for TTC that I found on the internet. I learned a lot about trying to have a baby and all that was involved. After several months had went by, we started using Ovulation Predictor Kits to see if that would help. I based Jadie's frustration in Chapter 7 on my own frustration over not even being able to get a positive on one of those. After several months in I went through a denial period where I told myself "oh this month didn't count because of this or because of that" or I wasn't counting my cycle days correctly so we weren't trying on just the right days and so on. My desire for children seemed to multiply around that time and grow very strong. I decided to share what was going on with us with my group of online friends. Several of my friends there had been through infertility and understood and all of them were so amazing to me over the next year and several months. Not long after that I found what I felt was my "theme" song which is the song I mention in Chapter 12 by Kellie Coffee. I would watch that video and bawl my eyes out. It was a very painful time, but feeling like other people had been where I was and understood was one of the only things that brought me comfort. For a very long time my husband remained strong and encouraged me. I remember him telling me often while holding me, "It'll happen." and I would always ask, "But how do you know?" and he would say he just did. He did a great job of hiding whatever he was going through and only showing it to me at times when I could handle it. After awhile it caught up to him and I would say both of us experienced the same level of pain through this experience. After a year had passed I knew from my TTC group and my research that we now had an automatic infertility diagnosis. It was a very difficult thing to face. I felt so stunned by it because I just figured it would never happen to me. Before we went through all this I had never even given it a whole lot of thought. That was a staggering and difficult landmark we had hit, but I would say the second year was even harder. We went back and forth between wanting to try something else to help like charting or consider going to the Doctor to wanting to just back off thinking about it so much and just let things happen when they did because of the emotional pain and stress it was causing us. One day I was sharing my heart with my dear friend Beth and was telling her about how we decided to just pray and try to be relaxed about things and try to not think about it so much for both of our sakes (just to try to have a break from thinking about it so much so maybe it wouldn't hurt as badly), but that there was one thing I wanted to look into before I forgot. I believe it was that same day that I researched something I had just heard about on my TTC group that I thought sounded like something I may have (since by this time I knew when I ovulated and about how my cycles tended to go). I researched it and was nearly positive that I had luteal phase defect. Most women who have this do not make enough progesterone and they tend to ovulate late in the cycle and once they've ovulated the second phase (luteal phase) of the cycle is quite short. Since the progesterone production is low, it does not line the uterus as it should so even if an egg is fertilized, the body does not sustain the pregnancy but releases the baby when the period starts causing an early miscarriage. (There are variations to this as well. Some women have irregular cycles with this and some Dr's believe women with this have a "weak" ovulation and the women are put on prescriptions to help give them a "stronger" ovulation, etc.) The bad news if I had that problem was that I had probably lost babies along our journey of trying to start a family. The good news was that it was so simple to treat. We struggled with when to go to a fertility specialist due to a few factors in our lives including finances. When do you dive in and go for it and have faith and when are you practical and try to be smart about things? Where is the line? We decided to wait a bit to go to the Doctor and to try to further "prove" that I was indeed ovulating but did have the LPD, I decided to start charting. So we took a break from trying (so that if I did have LPD we would not get pregnant and lose the baby without the proper medication) and I charted for three cycles. We decided to "take the plunge" and got a reference from my regular doctor to see a fertility specialist. We went at the end of January, 2009. I took along my charts and the other information I had from when I had taken OPK's and how short my luteal phase had always been. Since my temperatures on my chart and the OPK's showed in two ways that I ovulated, I felt confident that she would agree I had the LPD and we could get some answers or hopefully get moving forward. We talked to the specialist extensively and she looked over my charts (which she said saved her tons of time and questions) and we discussed many things. She did ask if I'd ever felt I was pregnant and we talked in detail about why and different things that had went on with my body those times and she said she was nearly positive I'd been getting pregnant and having early miscarriages. She asked me how many cycles I thought that had happened and I believe I told her four or five times. We were incredibly blessed because instead of confirming the LPD with testing as she said she normally did, she said the information I'd given her and the charts made it clear I had it. She said there could be more wrong, but she would give us a chance and give us 3 months worth of prometrium (bio-identical progesterone tablet you take orally from the day after ovulation on to help sustain a pregnancy). She said she didn't want to "put all our eggs in one basket," so she'd only give us 3 months but if that didn't work we would go back for further testing (which for me was first to check to see if my tubes were clear and my husband would have to have a sperm analysis done and we would keep going on testing from there for me). We felt so grateful for the chance and hoped we would get pregnant in that amount of time and would not have to go back for further testing. I was very excited to have at least one answer and be moving forward after all the months of doubt, wondering, questions, and uncertainty. However, realizing for sure that I did have LPD brought with it some sadness as I knew I had lost babies and wasn't even sure how many there had been. We ended up having enough prometrium to last us five months due to how many pills came with each "month" worth of prescription. I did take one month off for my own sanity and also to try to lose some weight. While I was glad the prometrium did it's job and was grateful to have something to help me keep a baby should I get pregnant, the symptoms and side effects it gave me were tricky and extensive. It gave me pregnancy symptoms and each month the symptoms grew more intense. It was very hard to not be able to trust my own body and the signs it was giving me and also very difficult to experience false hope especially after all the months of failed attempts. The month off did me some good and when we realized we had enough pills for the fifth cycle, I was excited but it felt like there was some pressure on us too. If this didn't work we'd be back to wondering what was going on, doctors appointments, uncomfortable tests, and possibly expensive treatments. Luckily for me the last few months God had given me an incredible, unearthly peace and I was able to endure those few last difficult months. The last month I felt I dealt with very well. Justin however was struggling some of the hardest he had been all along. It had been a very long and painful journey for us both. On August 10th we hit the two year mark of trying to have a baby. I have not gone into much detail on how we felt and a big part of that is simply because of how difficult it is to put into words. But here is part of what I journaled that day and I sum up some of the emotions we'd been going through:

"It has been two long years to the exact day since we have been TTC. In some ways I can't believe it has been that long. In some ways, the time has absolutely flown. In other ways, it does feel like FOREVER that we've wanted this sooo badly, but it eludes us. Like there is this wall between us and our greatest wish, hope, and dream but we don't know what it is, how to penetrate it, or how to make it go away so we can get to where we're trying to go. I remember distinctly sitting on our bed two years ago today reading my Bible together. We read many passages on parenting, prayed together, and talked about our hopes and dreams for our future baby/children. I remember feeling like it was one of the most exciting, meaningful, and overwhelmingly "big" days of my entire life. We were getting ready to start a family. What could be more wonderful or exciting than that? ... We had always said we would wait 4-5 years so as to have plenty of time just the two of us, etc. Now it is nearly our five year anniversary (beginning of next month) and still we have love in our hearts to give, but **are**

left with empty arms and crushed dreams. We have went through many phases throughout these two years. Especially me. I went through trying to convince myself nothing was wrong, getting beyond stressed and thinking of it constantly and worrying, denial and trying to come to some sort of peace with the whole thing and rely on God, to frantic-nearly-panicked-horrible-stress-and-worry-obsessing-mind-never-stopping-wondering-if-I-was-dreaming-up-symptoms-or-had-gone-crazy-willing-to-try-anything-and-everything-desperate-for-answers-crazy-mode, to feeling like I was gonna be okay, to not being able to decide where do you draw the line between being smart financially and trusting God, to taking the plunge in going to the doctor, to feeling like we finally had an answer and a simple solution and getting false hope that it would happen now, to utter frustration and despair at the horrific side effects of prometrium (including every symptom in the book and even swelling in my tummy which made me look and feel pregnant only to have it snatched away when AF reared her ugly head yet again), to anger . . . even at God and at the end of my rope and beyond all frustration, and finally to God giving me this AMAZING and WONDERFUL and much-needed peace. Now I am just kind of resigned. I'm tired of trying to find the balance of not having my hopes up and hoping. I'm just kind of hoping realizing that it may or may not happen any time soon. It still hurts, but I'm sooo glad to have all that junk behind me . . . I could make this much longer detailing all of the emotional and marital and spiritual ramifications of what we've been through, but I won't. It hurts . . . it sucks . . . but it just is. This is where we are. I'm okay with it. Again, it still hurts, but God will get us through. I think it has brought me closer to God and it has brought Justin & I closer together. I keep praying that God will teach us what He wants us to know, that we will get through this trial still honoring Him the way I know He wants us to. And I am still working on my book and want to use this for Him to bring Him honor and glory and also to help others through it which I'm sure is part of His plan and purpose. We still want to be parents more than anything. But this has helped us grow as people, as a couple, and as Christians trying to plug through this mire that has threatened to discourage us, bring us down, and choke us to death. I'm glad that God has thinned the mire for me and I can now feel solid ground beneath my feet. I don't know how to put into words how I can feel better (as in not so stressed or frantic or worried or obsessing), but still hurt over it at the same time. I feel at peace and ready to face what I must, but still hoping I won't have to. I don't know if that makes sense, but I have done my best to explain it. We have much to be grateful for in our lives and I will continue to praise Him for all He's done. I just hope and pray that our deepest heart desire is fulfilled soon.

I am starting my prometrium today since I ovulated yesterday. Soon (all too soon) I will have to take a pregnancy test. I HATE doing it. I cannot count the number of negatives I've had and I'm nearly beyond hoping at all that I will see that +. I try to hope beforehand, but whenever I take them it's so hard to dare to dream that I could ever see such a wonderful symbol representing what I long for so desperately with my entire being. Now it's back to the roller coaster of pregnancy symptoms, but knowing I cannot trust my body at all, but have to know that it's just the stupid pills doing their thing. And then . . . taking that test. I have been praying soo hard this month. I keep telling God I BELIEVE and have COMPLETE FAITH that He CAN do this, it's just if He will choose to that I can't know and that causes me to be sad and doubt. How interesting though that I ovulated the day before the 2 year anniversary and that we would find out very shortly before our 5 year wedding anniversary if it did indeed work this month. Humanly speaking the timing is perfect. But God may have other plans . . . I just don't know. And it's that not knowing that has been challenging and may continue to be for months . . . even years longer.

Here's to 2 years of infertility . . . of a thing that I thought would never happen to us but has. I have learned a lot and gone through quite a journey. I just pray it's over soon. Not b/c I don't feel I could handle more, but b/c I want it soo badly and it would be so awesome if it would happen now . . .

. . . Two Years . . . wow, two years. How much longer, I wonder?"

Just eleven days later, we got our positive pregnancy test on Friday, August 21st, 2009. Here are some snippets from what I journaled that day:

"So . . . I did it. I took the pregnancy test. I got up early before I had to get ready for work and I took it. Since I was still kind of sleepy, I didn't allow myself to go through the horrible emotions I normally associate with the dumb things, lol. I just took it, left it on the counter and came here to write this. I did glance at it before I left and I have to admit, I was a little surprised by what I saw there. But you never know, I'll give it the full amount of time and see what happens.

So much is resting on this. Humanly speaking the timing is great: our 2 year anniversary of trying was this month, it's almost our 5 year anniversary, if we were to get pregnant now we won't have to go and do the next tests at the infertility doctor. It was our last shot to not have to.

I have still had that indescribable peace. But yesterday I didn't want to test all that bad today but I know I needed to. When I told Justin I was going to, he said, "Don't test tomorrow!" When I asked him why he couldn't put it into words. I said, "Is it b/c it's easier to go on waiting b/c you know there's still a slight chance, but if I test, it's over?" and he said yes. My feelings exactly!

. . . A lot of this journey has been about "answers." Wanting them, not getting them, waiting for them, frustrated b/c we don't know them, etc. The other day it hit me. This month we are going to get an answer in a way. Not the kind we typically think of (like knowing why or what else is wrong and how to fix it), but the kind that God gives. This month we will find out if God has said, "Here is your miracle, it's over" or "I have My plans for you, keep waiting."

… *The result is* …

POSITIVE! I saw a PLUS SIGN. Something I was beginning to wonder if I'd ever see! I walked to the bathroom, hung onto the door frame for support, took some deep breaths and I prayed that I would accept whatever God had for me. I walked over to it with a bit of dread and made myself look at it right away. My heart nearly jumped out of my chest!!! I instantly began crying and saying out loud, "I'm pregnant" … "I'm pregnant" … "I'm pregnant" over and over in between gasping and crying. But not like a statement, but like a question, LOL … dropped to my knees on our bedroom floor and just kept telling Him "Thank You. Thank You sooo much! Thank You. I will tell everyone what You've done. Thank You."

… *God is sooooooo good (and that is WAYYY an understatement)* …"

I didn't understand why I had to go through that while I was and it was at times very agonizing and painful. But now I would not change that experience for the world. I feel I will always carry the scars of infertility on my heart, but it has helped shape me and my relationship with my husband and God very much. I also feel I cherished my pregnancy and now my time as a mother so much more and am much more grateful than I would have been. Not that I still wouldn't have enjoyed those things, but it's just deeper and more meaningful for me I believe. I also wouldn't have my sweet Jenna had it happened at a different time and I would not trade her for anything! Things happened as they were meant to and when they were meant to and I can see a lot of good that God brought about now looking back on it. I also believe God allowed me to go through it so I could help other women and even couples. I feel honored to be able to do that and I am very passionate about this book as I feel it is a huge step in that direction.

While I was writing this book, we began trying to have our second baby. We went back to the OB we had used while I was pregnant with Jenna to get my prescription for prometrium and we started trying in May of 2011. My doctor gave me four months worth of medicine and said that if we didn't become pregnant during that time, that we would "go from there." Thank goodness the prometrium didn't have near the side effects the second time around as it did the first. We ended up having enough medicine for five cycles. So we took July off and finished up the medicine in October and were still not pregnant. So we made an appointment to go back to the doctor and we weren't sure what would happen from there. If she'd let us try other treatments or if we would be getting testing done since we never had to before getting pregnant with Jenna. At the beginning of this second journey I found fears creeping up already and was having thoughts of wanting to beg God to not let me go through what we did last time again. I was afraid to go through infertility again or never have another child at all. I was so grateful for Jenna and I would not have been angry if we couldn't have more, but I would have had to mourn that as I would have been heartbroken. But after a couple of months of having those fears I stopped beating myself up for having those feelings and realized that it was understandable after what we'd went through the last time. Once I accepted that, I released those feelings and found peace in waiting in the Lord's will again. The journey didn't seem to drag at all like I had thought it might. And this time by the time we reached the point that we knew we were going to the doctor, I was no longer afraid of it like I had been the last time or at the beginning of this time. I knew that it was in God's hands and it would all be okay. I was also ready to find out if something else was wrong and was no longer nervous of tests that I knew would be uncomfortable and painful and have more times of waiting and possible treatments and so on. So we were just calmly awaiting the day of our appointment in mid-December. So we didn't try in the November cycle because I didn't have my medicine and we didn't want to risk miscarriage if we did conceive. Sometime around Thanksgiving I started having symptoms pop up and I kept getting more and more. I blamed some on having a cold and others on the fact that my body must still be having after effects from the prometrium of some sort. Finally I had so many and some that couldn't be blamed on anything that Justin and I were really beginning to wonder. He told me I should test just in case I had somehow gotten pregnant so I could start my medicine right away. I looked at my chart (since I'd been doing that again for me and my Dr. to keep track of everything) and made a mental note to test a day or two later since I would be about ten days past ovulation at that point. To say I was extremely shocked when the test said "pregnant" on December 2nd would be an understatement. It was just so highly unlikely! I got on my medicine right away and my symptoms continued. To say that Justin and I were thrilled would also be an understatement. I felt so incredibly blessed to have yet another miracle on the way! What a wonderful early Christmas present! Our next appointment with our Dr. to take the next steps ended up being our first OB appointment. Since I got on my medicine late, my Dr. wanted to see if there "was even a heartbeat" or if the pregnancy was "even viable." We did an ultrasound and I was not surprised, but very grateful to the Lord, to see a heartbeat and everything measuring right on track! And so we received our second miracle baby. I guess God wanted to make sure He got all the glory and He certainly did/does! For the record, I believe God is the only creator of life medicine and/or treatment or no. But I guess He just wanted to make extra sure in this case and that's just fine with me! So I just wanted to continue to share my story to give comfort and encouragement to those who are maybe trying to have another baby after going through infertility and also since I'd already shared our journey in that area thus far. I also wanted to again make sure I did my part to tell people what He has done for me.

♥ ♥ ♥

Even though I have experienced this myself and knew the experiences, thoughts, and feelings of the women on my group, I still wanted to make sure I got an extremely accurate picture of all these women have been through and accuracy on the different causes they faced for not being able to conceive. So I sent out a detailed interview to a few who were willing to participate. I wanted to name you here and thank you for opening up and sharing to help others. Ashleigh Schemenaur, Melissa Carswell, Brieanne Robson, and Melissa Reiner.

Infertility is a very personal and emotional thing to go through. For me personally, it has been one of the biggest trials I have ever had to face. But I wanted to encourage all of you who have been through it or are going through it to be understanding of one another. Everyone is different and will try to tackle this in different ways. Some people will want to chart and some won't. Some will not want to pursue any medical treatment, some will want to pursue it to a certain extent, and some will go as far as possible to conceive themselves. Some will want to adopt (or do a combination of that and continuing to try for biological children) and some will decide to stop trying to have children at all. I just ask that you all remember that we are all different and to accept how other feel about it, respect each other's decisions, and continue to support and encourage one another. I have found that most people going through infertility tend to be very understanding of other's decisions in this area. If you have not been through it personally, I hope that you will try to open your mind as far as treatment goes if you feel negative towards it or against it. Infertility is no different than anything else that can go wrong with any part of your body and at times it requires treatment if the couple so chooses.

You may have noticed that I left things rather open ended with Haden and Gracie. There is a reason for that and I'm very excited to share more about them in a future novel. You can also expect to read more on Amy, Jadie, Emma, Kendra and their families as well.

Feel free to write me at *sallymjoneswrites@gmail.com* or follow me on Facebook: *www.facebook.com/sallymjoneswrites.*

Lastly, I just want to say that I am so glad that I have finished this project. It is so exciting for me to be publishing my first book! I know some people may not like it or may not like my writing, but that's not important. I am not claiming to be an excellent writer, but I pray that I accomplished my goal of touching people's hearts and helping and encouraging them. And I followed what I felt God wanted me to do. I also kept my promise to Him. Lord, I have told everyone I possibly can in the best way I can think of, what You've done for me. To God be the glory for this book and for all He's done in all of our lives.

Love in Christ,

Sally M Jones

CPSIA information can be obtained at www.ICGtesting.com
Printed in the USA
BVOW011202040213

312320BV00002B/11/P

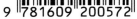